HOT BODIES, COOL STYLES
NEW TECHNIQUES IN SELF-ADORNMENT

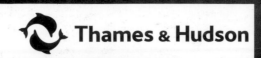
Thames & Hudson

HOT BODIES, COOL STYLES
NEW TECHNIQUES IN SELF-ADORNMENT

TED POLHEMUS

Photographs by **UZi PART B**

Practical advice section by Betti Marenko

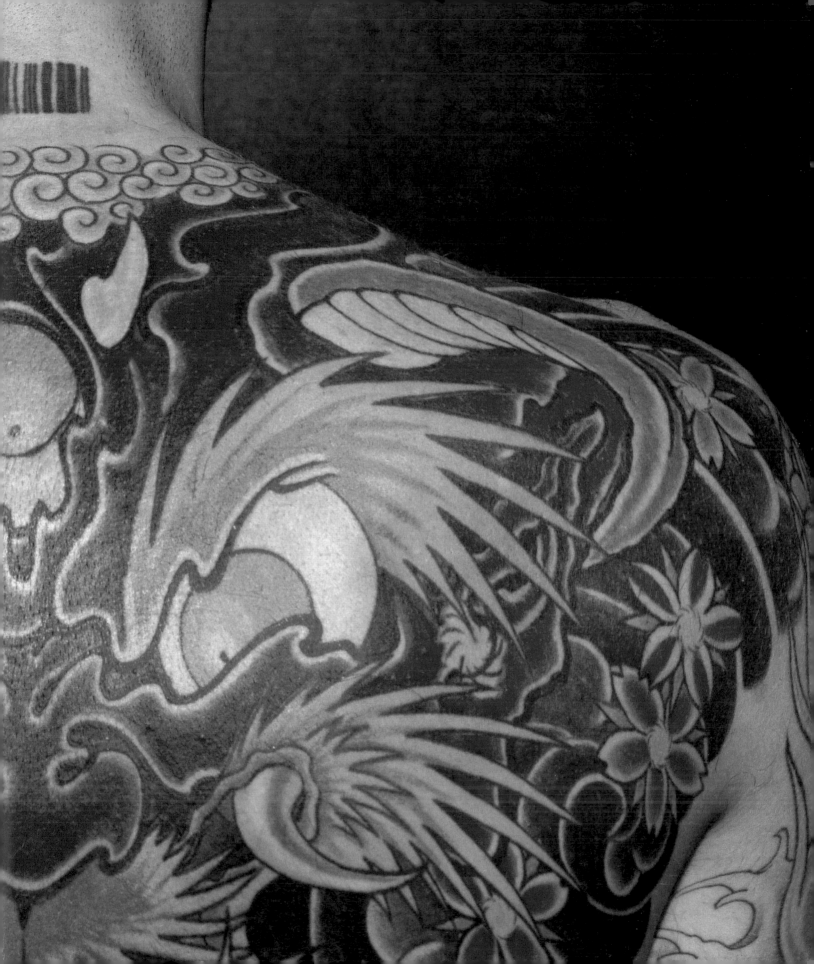

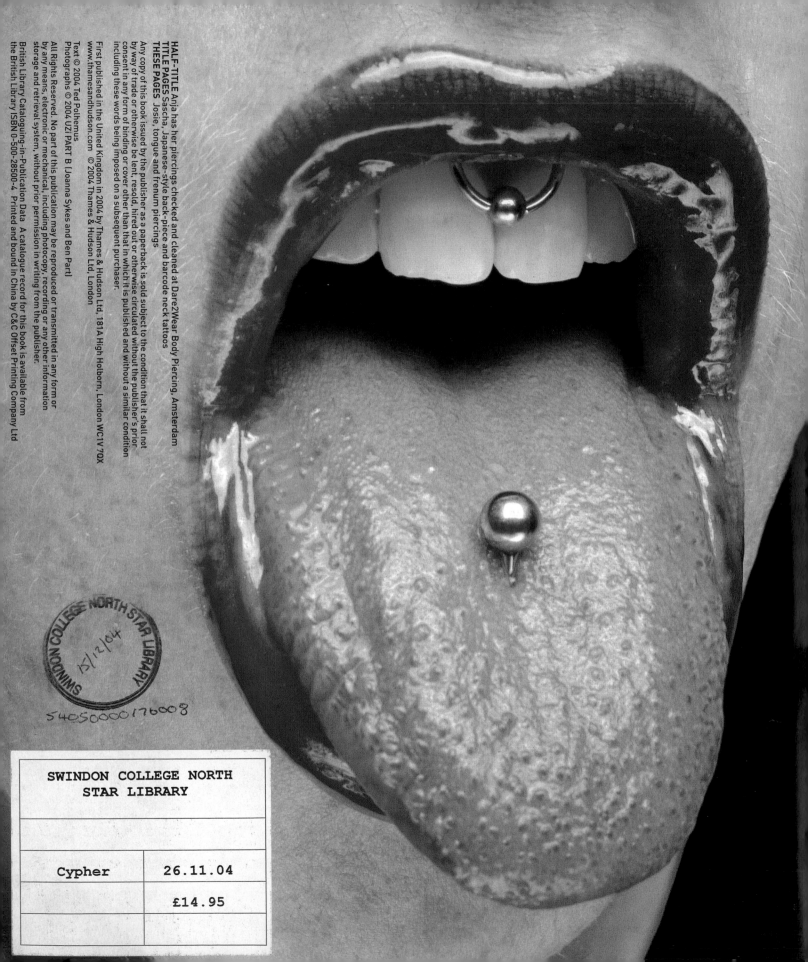

HALF-TITLE Anja has her piercings checked and cleaned at Dare2Wear Body Piercing, Amsterdam
TITLE PAGES Sascha. Japanese-style back-piece and barcode neck tattoos
THESE PAGES Josie, tongue and frenum piercings

Any copy of this book issued by the publisher as a paperback is sold subject to the condition that it shall not by way of trade or otherwise be lent, resold, hired out or otherwise circulated without the publisher's prior consent in any form of binding or cover other than that in which it is published and without a similar condition including these words being imposed on a subsequent purchaser.

First published in the United Kingdom in 2004 by Thames & Hudson Ltd, 181A High Holborn, London WC1V 7QX
www.thamesandhudson.com

© 2004 Thames & Hudson Ltd, London

Text © 2004 Ted Polhemus
Photographs © 2004 UZI PART B (Joanna Sykes and Ben Part)

All Rights Reserved. No part of this publication may be reproduced or transmitted in any form or by any means, electronic or mechanical, including photocopy, recording or any other information storage and retrieval system, without prior permission in writing from the publisher.

British Library Cataloguing-in-Publication Data A catalogue record for this book is available from the British Library ISBN 0-500-28500-4 Printed and bound in China by C&C Offset Printing Company Ltd

CONTENTS

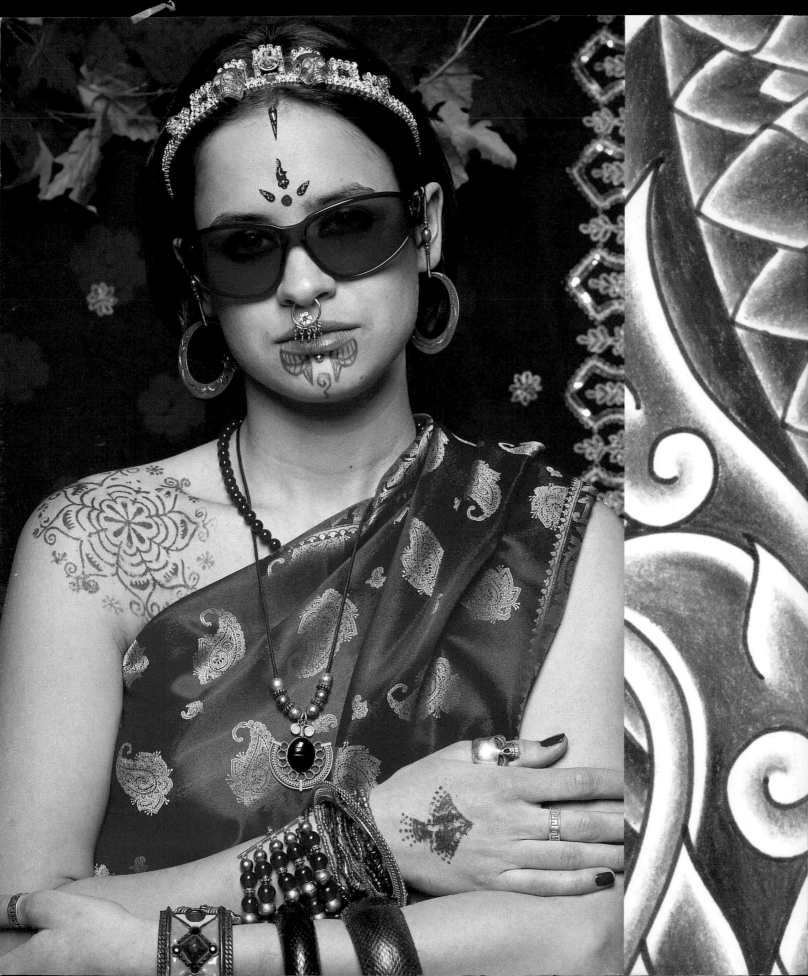

INTRODUCTION

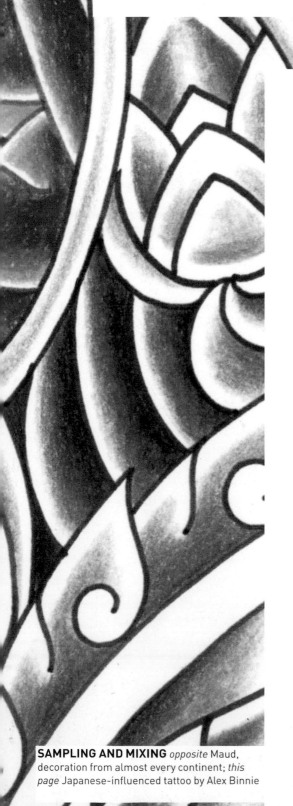

The human body is so bland and unexciting. We cannot compete with the striking graphic dynamics of the zebra, the rococo flamboyance of the parrot, the hallucinogenic dazzle of a shoal of tropical fish or the subtle, textural variation of a leopard. Nor do our bodies undergo exciting visual transformations: no dramatic unfurling of the peacock's tail, no sudden shift of fluorescent pattern like that exhibited by the squid and, unlike most other primates, the backsides of ovulating human females don't turn lurid shades of pink. Just as we possess no natural weapons or protective armour, so too must we resort to techniques of our own invention in order to be visually striking.

The range and diversity, the inventiveness and daring of the different methods that humans have devised for altering their appearance is truly astounding – from the simple act of sticking flowers or leaves in the hair to the complexity of changing the shape of an infant's head, embedding precious stones in teeth, covering a body in intricate scarification designs or constructing a wig or a shell necklace. These techniques constitute a formidable body of human knowledge and innovation. Moreover, as most of them existed globally long before the Age of Exploration, we must conclude either that parallel experiments and discoveries occurred on separate continents or that they predate the geographic spread of our most ancient ancestors. Either way, such geographic diversity obliges us to accept the fundamental importance of body decoration for our species.

SAMPLING AND MIXING *opposite* Maud, decoration from almost every continent; *this page* Japanese-influenced tattoo by Alex Binnie

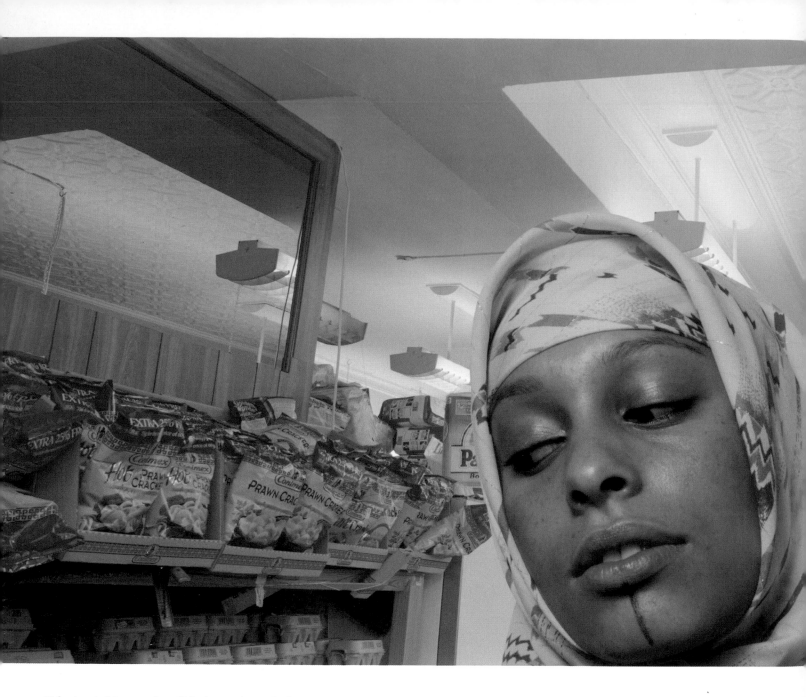

What might occasion this importance? There is now a general consensus among anthropologists that what set Homo sapiens apart from all other animals and gave our species predominance is an extraordinary capacity for symbolic thought. Typically, this mental facility has been equated with verbal language and the art that our ancestors left behind on the walls of caves and as sculpted objects. But as we increasingly recognize appearance as 'statement' – as we come to appreciate that our choices of appearance style have something to 'say' – we begin to see what traditional cultures have known all along: that right at the heart of this symbolic universe, which sets our species apart, is the art and the language of the styled, customized human body.

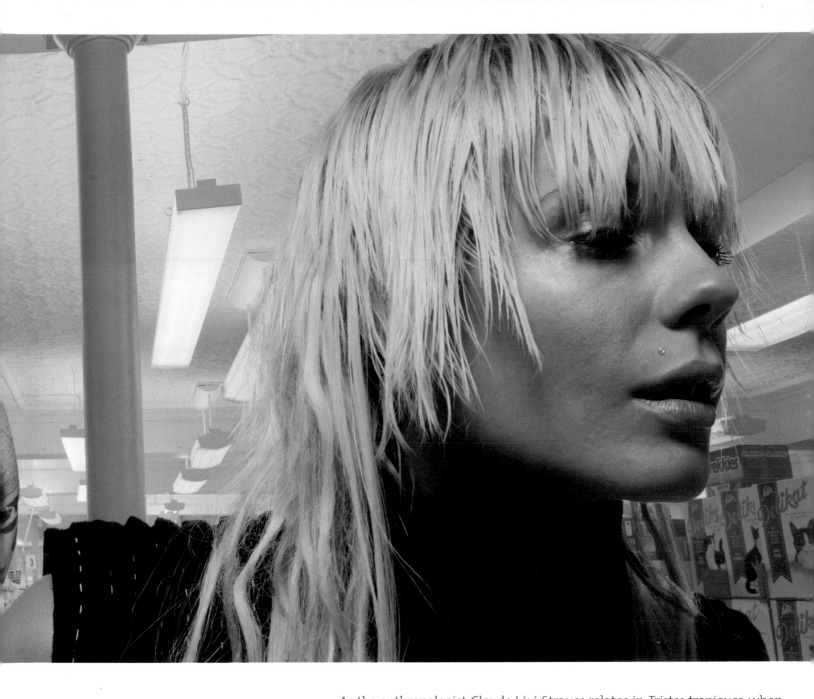

UNPRECEDENTED FREEDOM

exists today in choosing contrasting techniques and styles of body decoration. In the global 24/7 supermarket of style, fashion no longer dictates one look that all must follow, and each individual expresses – advertises – her- or himself by means of a distinctive appearance style. *Above* Grace, Netherlands, with Moroccan chin tattoo and Tory, Canada, with blue hair extensions

As the anthropologist Claude Lévi-Strauss relates in *Tristes tropiques*, when Western missionaries berated the Caduveo Indians of Brazil for 'wasting' so much time painting designs on their bodies the Indians responded indignantly: 'Why are you so stupid [that] you do not paint yourselves[...]?' The conclusion to be drawn is that 'To be a man it was necessary to be painted; to remain in the natural state was to be no different from the beasts'. By painting, tattooing, adorning, piercing and all sorts of other means, human beings bring their bodies into the symbolic universe. The human body is, by its very nature, special and essential – the one object we cannot do without, the one object that is also a subject – and therefore it stands at the centre of this symbolic universe.

If this brings us closer to understanding the motivation behind the development of all these extraordinary (often downright mind-boggling) techniques for transforming appearance, it also gives a clue as to why our physical bodies evolved into such visually inconspicuous and unexciting forms. Our skin is a blank canvas, waiting, as the Caduveo well knew, for the artist to perform his or her magic. But what a perfect canvas! Unlike the fur of our primate relations, our naked – blank – skin is an artistic medium offering almost unlimited possibilities for the many diverse techniques we shall explore in this book.

WHAT YOU LOOK LIKE
is no longer strictly determined by social situation and culture or even fashion. Free from rules, appearance is now a matter of personal creativity. *below* Cecilia designed her North Star belly tattoos to mimic those drawn on superstitious sailors (and later, their women) to guide them home; *opposite* a very different look sported at Carnival, Rotterdam

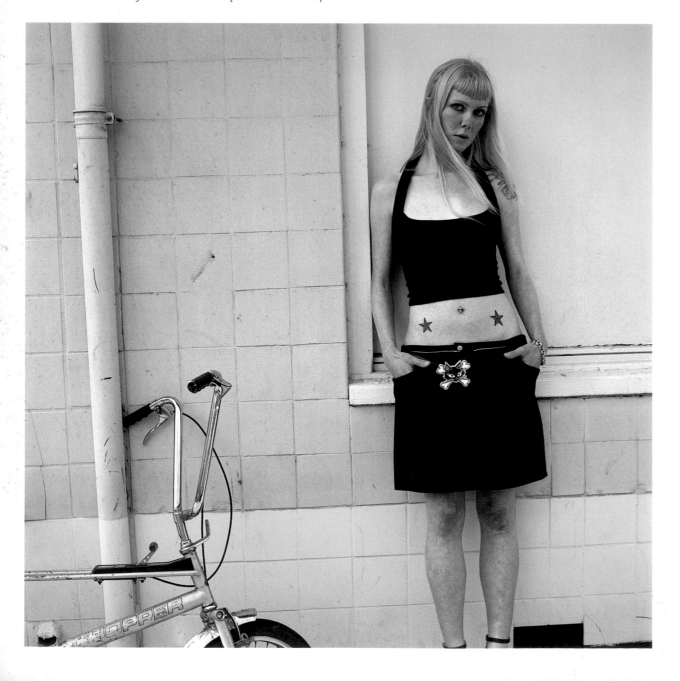

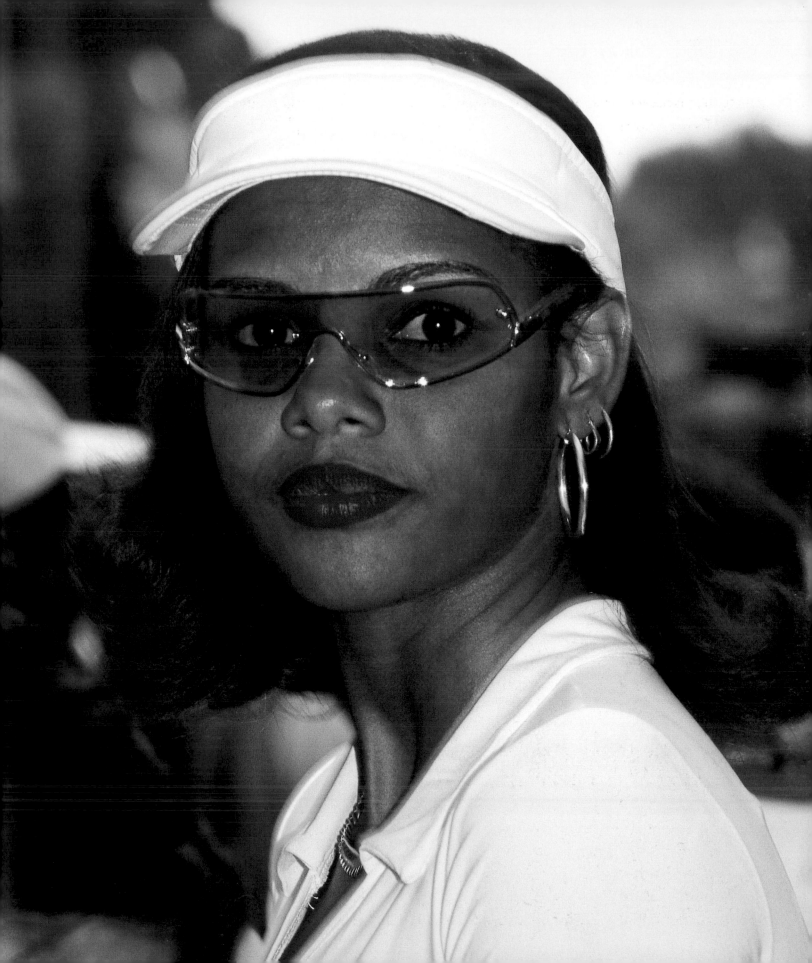

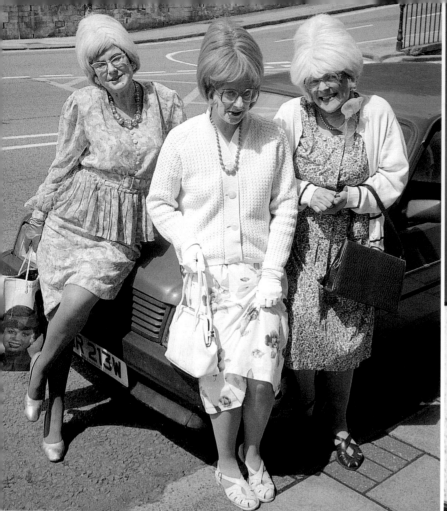

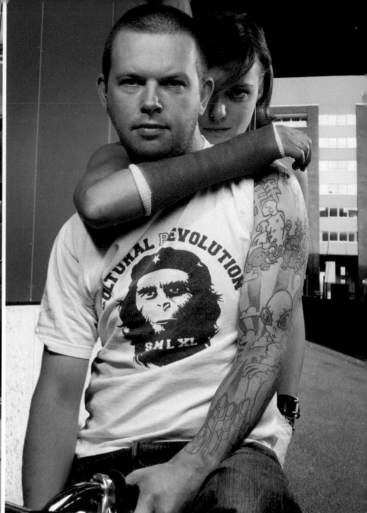

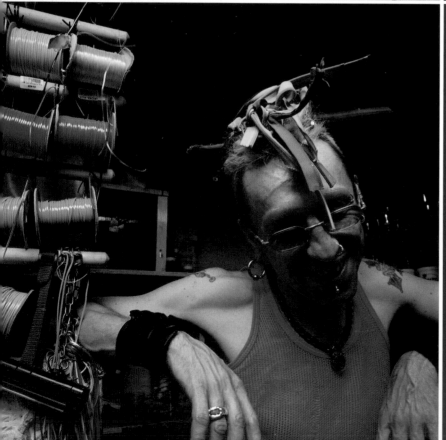

IDENTITY IN THE 21ST CENTURY

is primarily self-constructed. Within a world of diversity and difference, style has become a crucial, indispensable tool – a language system – for its expression. This is true of all aspects of style, from home decor to cars, kitchens to cuisine, but body style is undoubtedly our most powerful and effective means of signalling 'where we are at'. *clockwise from left* zips woven into hair at Pepi's Hairspace; Häf and friends from Natural Theatre in multi-coloured wigs and cardigans performing *Housewives*; *above* Stuart designed his tattoos, inked by Dan Gold at Kings Cross Tattooing, to mark a psychic event: 'my tattoos are about the unknown', and Natalie chooses red to decorate the plaster cast on her broken arm; *opposite* Sam, Carolien and Errol, a tattooed family at The Inkstitution; Karen shows the results of seven hours of work braiding and adding extentions at Emm & Bee's; Angelique at Admiraal Tattoo and her partner Peter; Riangeli and Marilia wear street-style sportswear and gold jewelry

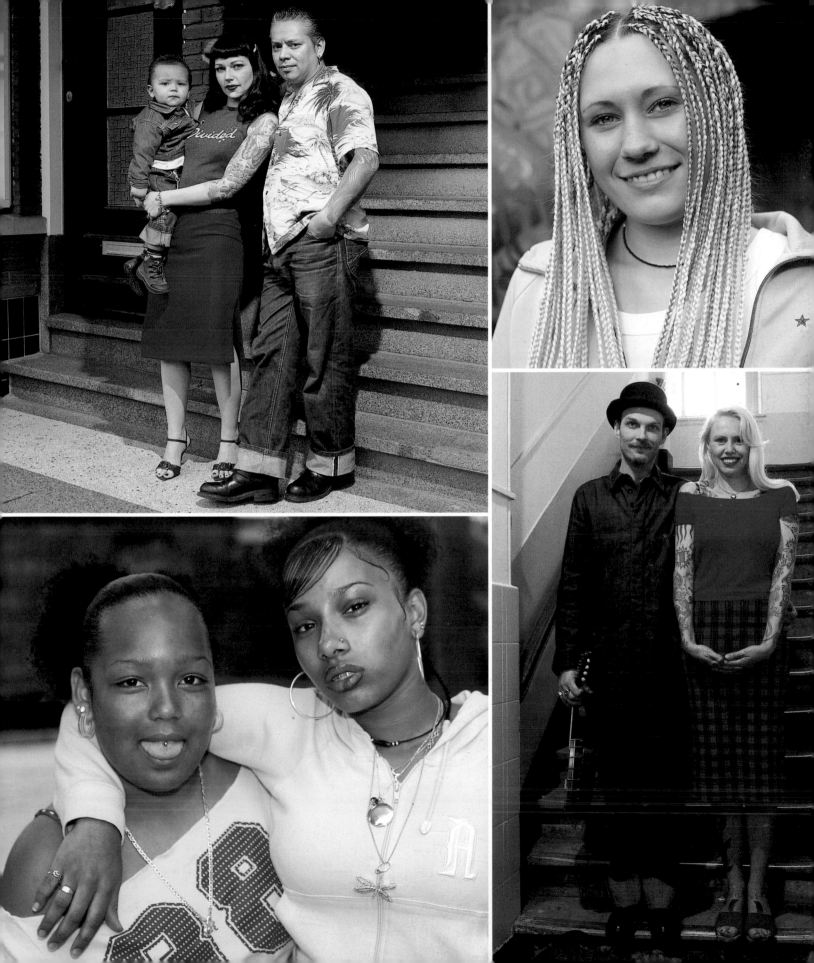

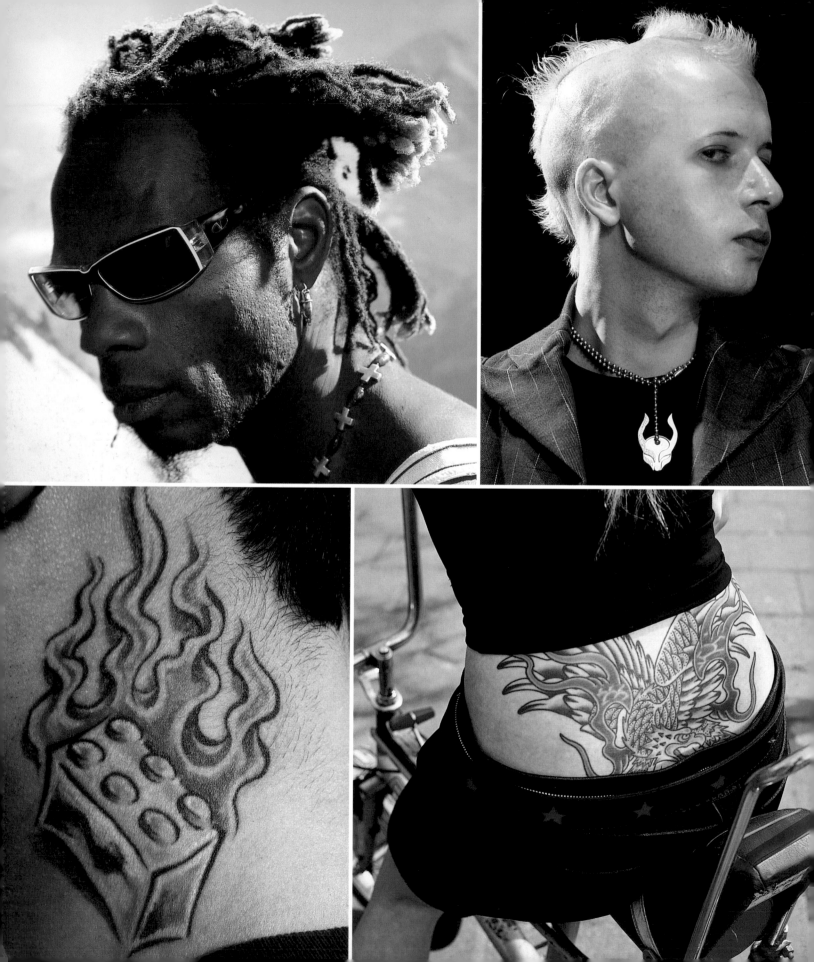

HUMAN SKIN AND HAIR ARE IDEAL MEDIA for creative expression. Surely it is no coincidence that the only species that deliberately, consciously and persistently transforms its appearance has evolved the perfect canvas for such body art? *opposite from top left, clockwise* Sam, Cameroon, bleached-tip dreads and designer sunglasses; Alex, UK, bleached fluffy Mohawk; Cecilia, Sweden, traditional Western sailor-style eagle tattoo by Rob Admiraal at Admiraal Tattoo; Giorgio, Italy, flaming Lego-block neck tattoo he designed to symbolize the 'click' with his girlfriend, inked by Gert at Tattoo Mania; *below* Sascha, Netherlands, with Rockabilly adornments including tattoos

So why, then, didn't we completely become the naked ape of Desmond Morris's famous phrase? Why, in other words, did we retain areas of fur that gradually got longer, becoming hair? Perhaps because hair too is a wonderfully transformable stylistic medium: you can do so much with it – colouring, cutting, razoring off or into designs, plaiting, sculpting into gravity-defying shapes and so on. To take this idea to its extreme, perhaps we developed hair so that we could have hairdressers, just as we became fur-less and naked to facilitate the body arts that use skin as their canvas.

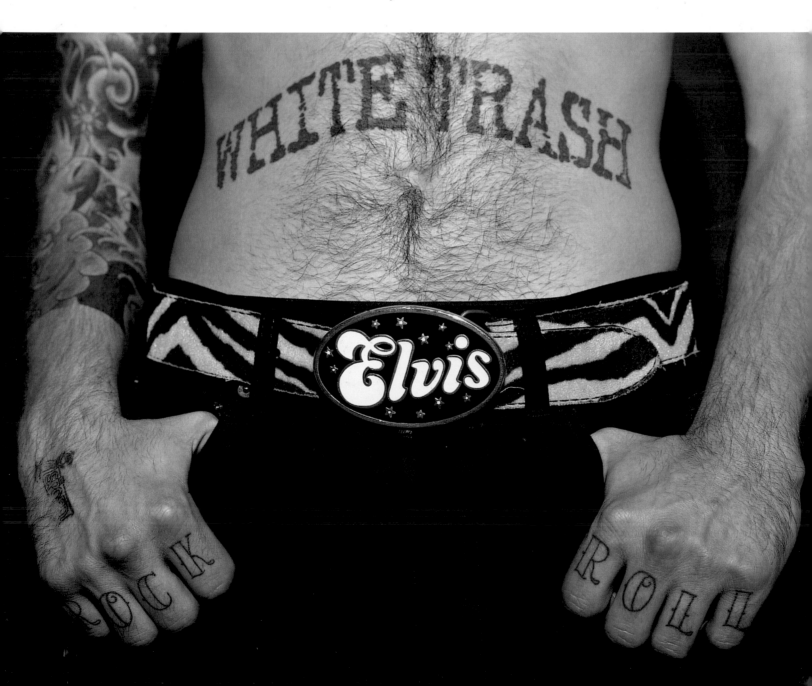

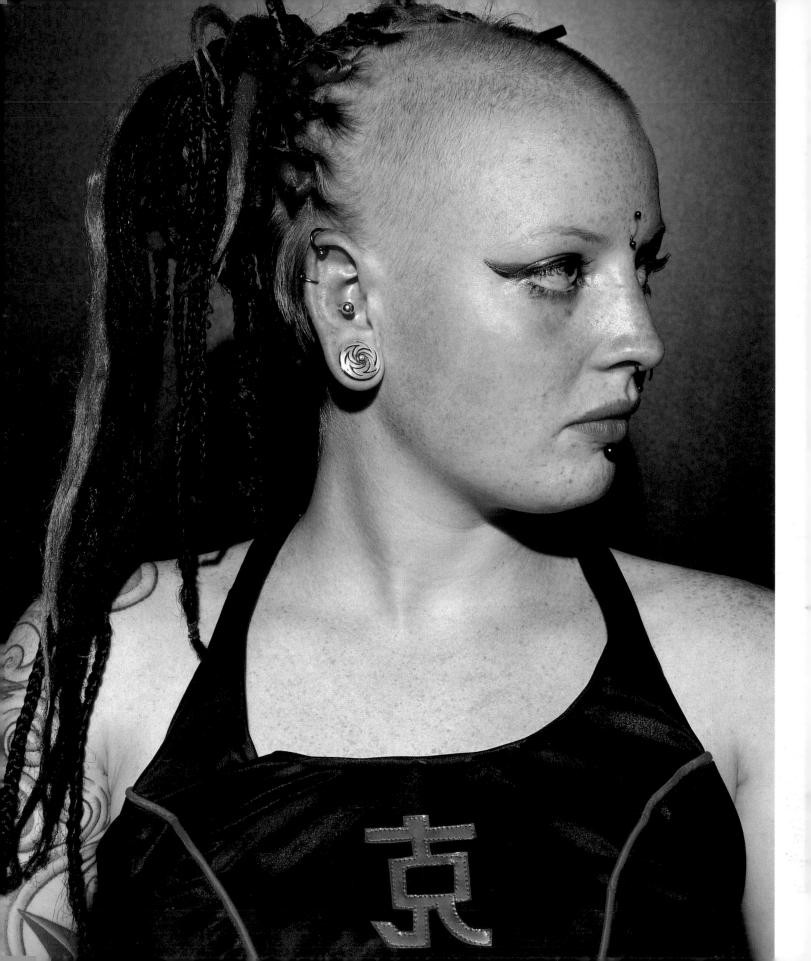

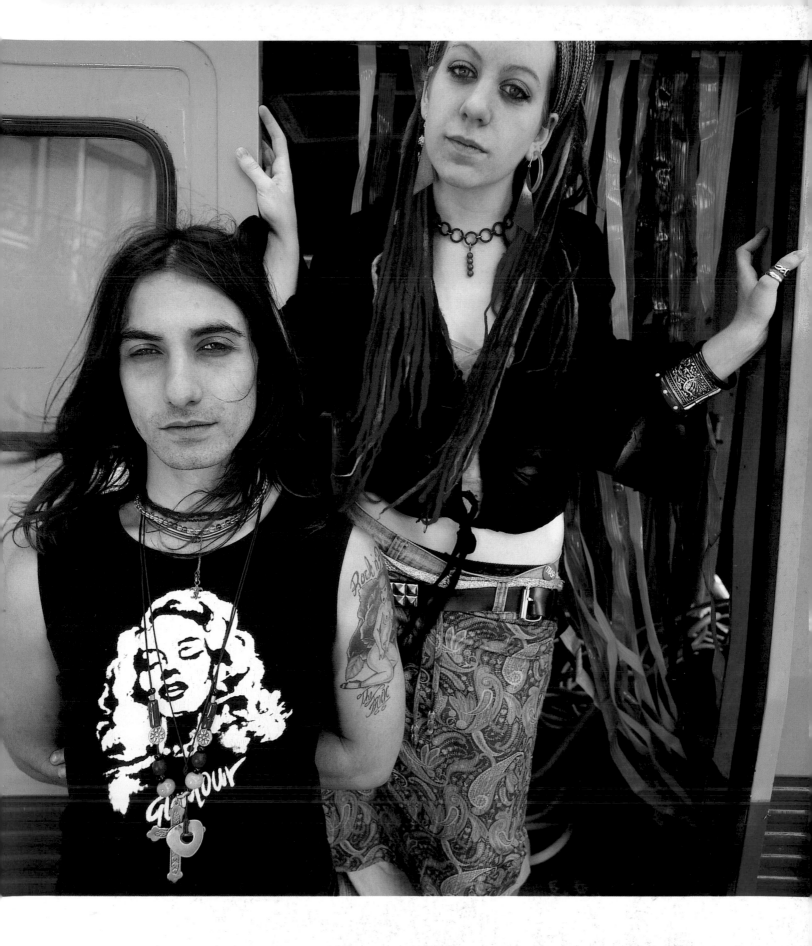

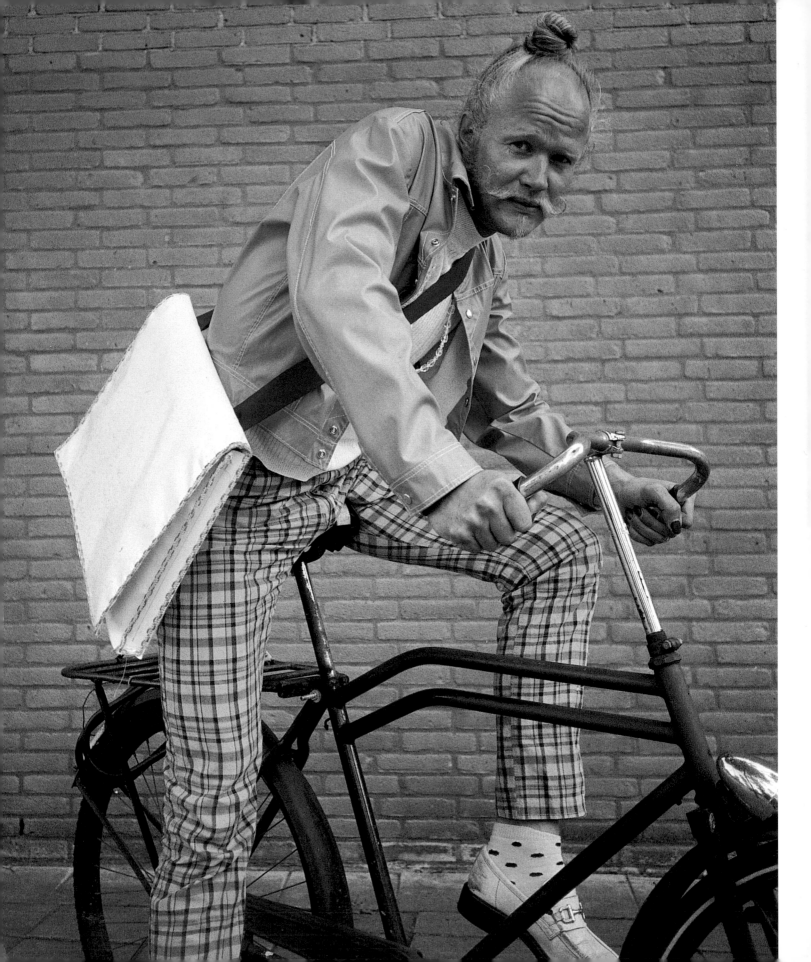

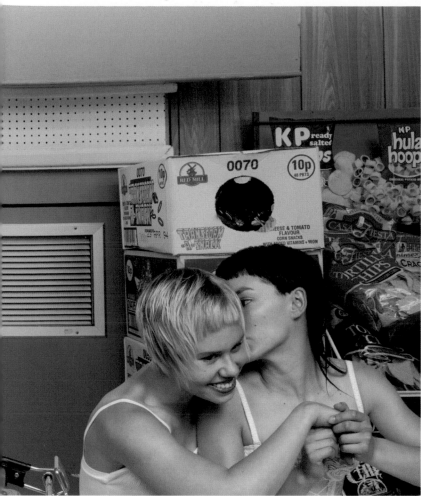

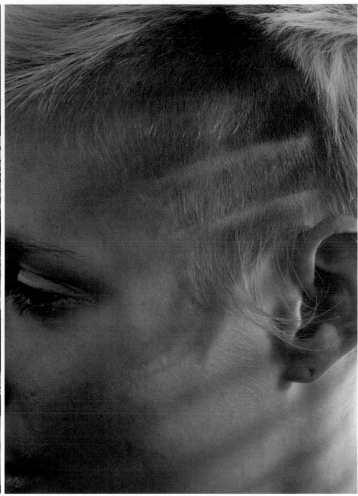

ALTHOUGH RESOLUTELY INDIVIDUALISTIC, some looks suggest subculture affiliations. But unlike, for example, the tattooed insignia of a particular group of Bikers, most do not explicitly proclaim membership of a particular 'tribe'. *previous pages* Noraly describes herself as a Cyberpunk; Rick and Jess might be seen as Hippies or Travellers, but prefer to avoid such labels. Jess: 'All my clothes, hair and accessories are just about adorning memories, stories or ideas on to the outside of my body as well as having them inside. It's about music but also art, books, politics, friends and family. How I look is the evidence of my history.'

HAIRSTYLE SIGNALS PERSONAL IDENTITY, lifestyle and values. *opposite* Pieter wears his hair in a bun with a handlebar moustache – a contemporary dandy or, as he says, a 'nowhereman'; *above* Elisa & Elisa use extensions and bleaching; *above right* Tory wears razor lines derived from hip hop culture and feathering from suedehead girls – a 'rock chick' hairdresser, her crosscultural experiments are influenced by her transatlantic lifestyle

From the very beginning (we know that Cro-Magnons decorated their bodies, both living and dead) our species marked itself out as the only decorated ape. (With one possible exception: recent evidence suggests that Neanderthals living in Europe at the same time as Homo sapiens made jewelry and painted their bodies.) Far from constituting a frivolous activity, as many in Western culture would automatically categorize anything to do with appearance, this served as a key medium of communication and symbolic representation. This is perfectly acknowledged in the word 'cosmetics', which comes from the Greek word *kosmos*, meaning order, universe and ornament. It is surely no coincidence, therefore, that as our ancestors made greater use of decoration, they gradually replaced their fur with the more creatively exploitable materials of skin and hair.

This was long ago. But as we review all the different, ancient techniques for transforming appearance, what is most fascinating is how many of these are available, coveted and now given new creative potential in our 21st-century supermarket of style.

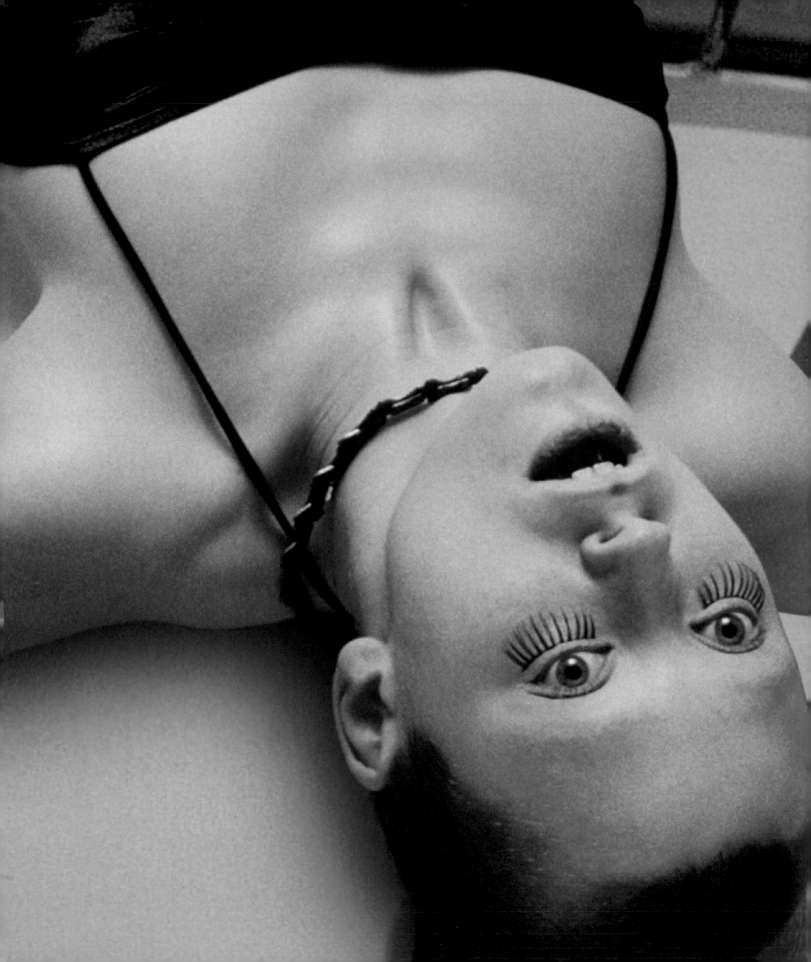

CHAPTER ONE

THE PAINTED BODY

No doubt body painting began by accident rather than design: stains on hands, feet or face caused by charcoal, berries or clay. But when the realization dawned that this effect could be controlled and the body marked deliberately – rendering it more attractive, more meaningful, a cultural rather than a natural object – body art was born. (And, arguably, art itself – for is it not likely that the first canvas was the most, literally, to hand?) It is impossible to know when this event actually took place but recent excavations on the South African coast have found seventy-thousand-year-old pieces of red ochre that it is believed were used for drawing designs on the body.

If the first such marks were made using only fingers, it would have been a simple step to the discovery that twigs, leaves or brushes made from animal fur could create particular effects and decorative styles. If the first pigments were simply those that were already to hand, the next step would have been the invention of technologies for making colours more intense, varied or long-lasting – for example baking or mixing with other substances. Over time, trade with neighbouring groups would have expanded the primitive palette. Reflections in water could have served as mirrors long before the same effect could have been produced using beaten metal or, later still, glass. But where difficulties in seeing your own body led to friends painting each other, this had the added advantage – like grooming in non-human primates – of reinforcing social bonds.

BODY PAINTING AS COMMUNICATION
opposite Barbara uses upside-down make-up for an upside-down street performance

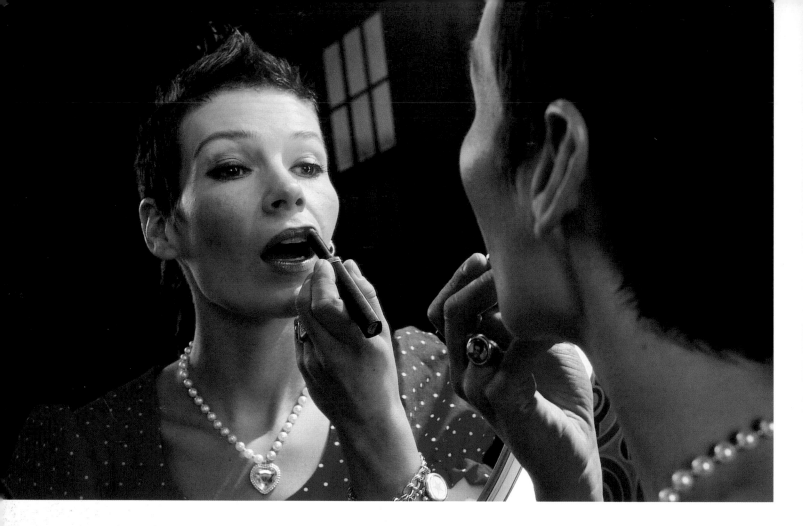

At first glance it seems a big jump from our ancestors' body painting to the gleaming laboratories of Revlon, Christian Dior, Max Factor, MAC and others where eyeshadows are created in every perceptible shade and a lipstick can be devised that doesn't smear even during the most passionate kiss. But the really significant differences between then and now are social and stylistic rather than technological.

Most obviously, what was once (at least in warm climates) an art that extended from head to toe has now been focused upon the face, in the form of cosmetics. There are exceptions (body painting at pop festivals, nightclub performers, carnival dancers), but it was inevitable that the advance of clothing and a more pervasive definition of modesty should bring a transition from body to face painting. (And, if the dictates of modesty are carried further to cover most of the face – as in many Muslim countries – painting focuses on the eyes, the feet and the hands.)

More interesting is the question of why cosmetics in Western culture have become so gender-specific, with 'real men', at most, restricted to natural-look preparations, which it is hoped will be invisible. Any quick glance through a

RECENT EVIDENCE SUGGESTS
that humans have been painting their bodies for at least 70,000 years. In the West, cosmetics have primarily focused on the face, accentuating and shaping natural features such as lips, eyes and cheekbones. *above* Nina, Norway, juxtaposes traditional red lipstick with less conventional Mohawk and dreads. *opposite* Majorie, Netherlands, steps outside the cosmetic tradition of the West – a dedicated Yogini and a street performer, she paints her face blue in tribute to the Lord Krishna

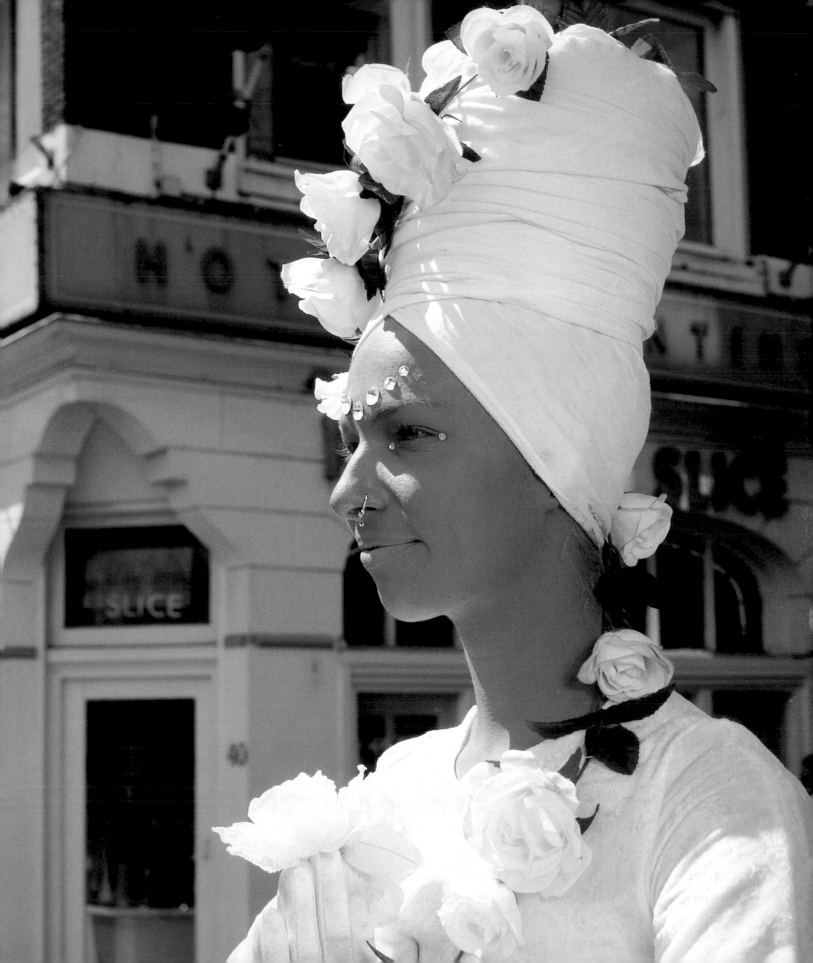

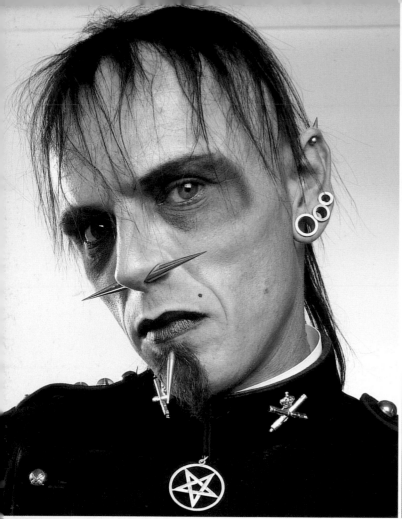

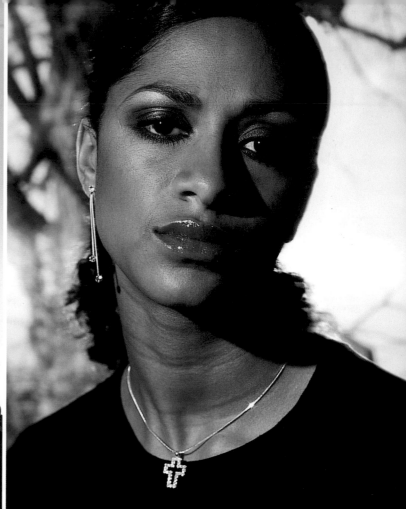

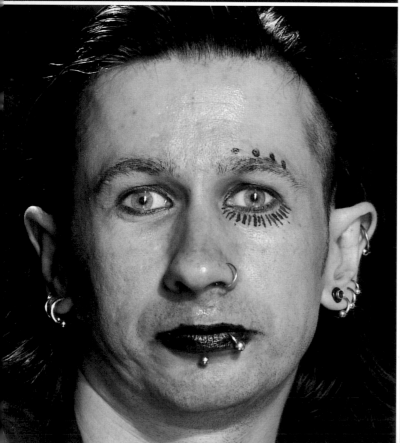

A MAN WEARING MAKE-UP,

even today, is seen as exceptional and challenging to mainstream definitions of masculinity. In tribal societies it was often the men who used body paint to demonstrate their peacock-like flamboyance, but in recent centuries make-up has been seen as an exclusively feminine body art. This presumption has been challenged by male Punks, New Romantics and Goths. *from left, clockwise* JG, Goth, uses black lipstick and eye make-up to delineate his features; Marcel's look, reminiscent of Marilyn Manson, is constructed using coloured contacts, piercings and dark make-up; Valesca *above* and Isabella *opposite right* present the conventional made-up, feminine face while *opposite* Lisa's more radical Cyberpunk look still uses make-up to highlight the features of the face

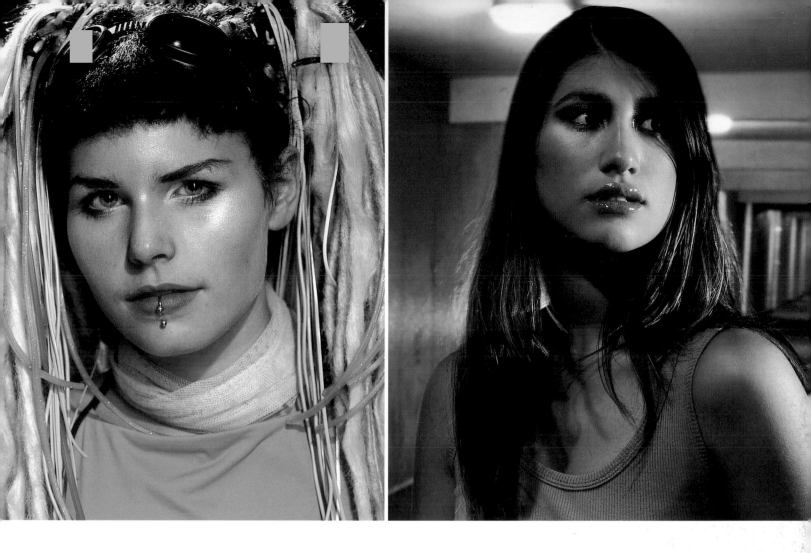

book on body decoration in ancient tribal societies shows that it is typically the men who exhibit the most extraordinary body painting. Even throughout much of European history, upper-class men used and often clearly delighted in cosmetics that loudly proclaimed their artifice.

In *The Psychology of Clothes*, the English writer J. C. Flugel identifies 'The Great Masculine Renunciation' of all forms of adornment for men, which intensified dramatically in the aftermath of the French Revolution. And he proposes – no doubt correctly – that this shift away from the colourful and the flamboyant came from the concern of the upper class to distance itself from extravagance and leisure in order to appear more socially responsible. (The loss of powders, extravagant wigs, lace and so forth being the price of keeping the revolution confined to France.) Subsequently, the Industrial Revolution (which brought a huge expansion of the hardworking, entrepreneurial and sartorially more restrained middle class) and the Age of Empire (which sharpened the distinction between unadorned 'superiority' and decorated natives) further reinforced

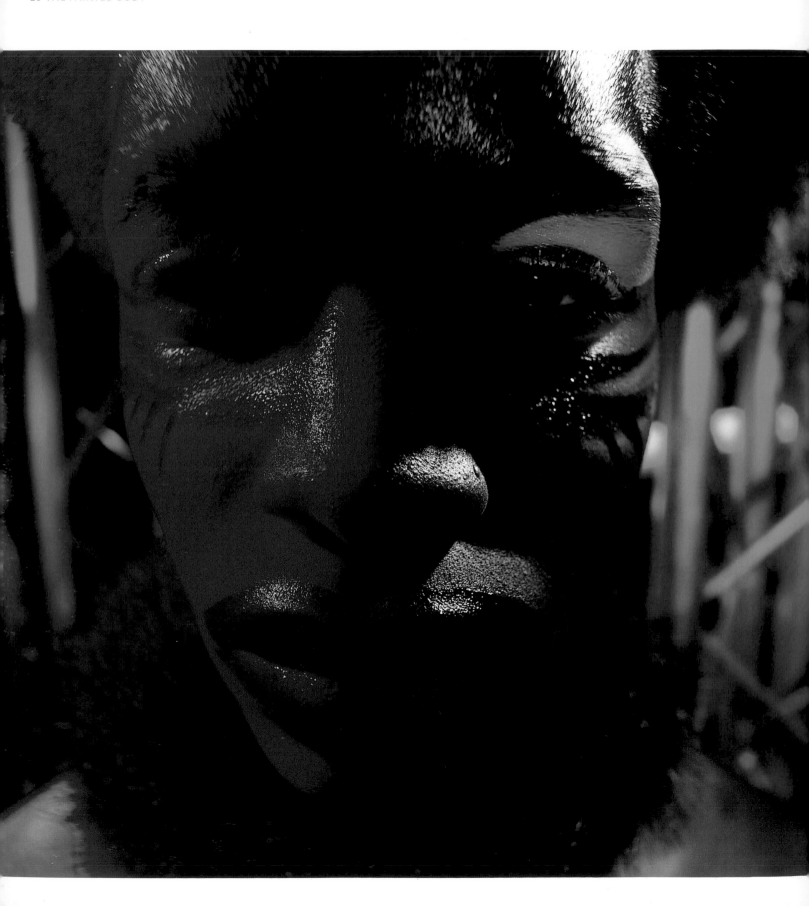

SKIN CAN BE USED AS A CANVAS,
without regard to natural features. When men paint
their faces or bodies, breaking free from the restricting
conventions accepted by most women, they often use
colour and design in a bold, graphic way that harks back
to the styles of tribal peoples. *opposite* Martin with face
painted in graphic style; beyond doubt, the most striking
development in contemporary body or face painting is
that found among male sports fans – *right* football fan
Jean-Luc-Dirk celebrates the French team

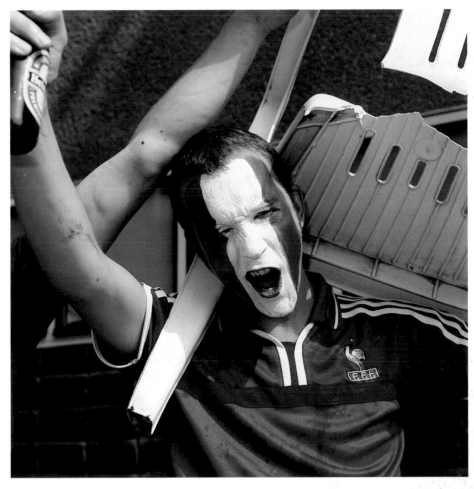

a Western definition of masculinity that excluded 'frivolous' adornment to
the point at which men became nearly invisible.

This presumption that real men don't use make-up has been remarkably
persistent. Although it often seemed in the 1970s and 1980s that Glam
Rockers, Punks, New Romantics and Goths would triumph over this taboo,
and despite perennial reports in the media announcing that a breakthrough
in cosmetics for men is imminent, we find that lipstick, eyeshadow, mascara
and any other visible cosmetics remain fully within the territory of 'feminine'
adornments.

Yet, at the same time, a new form of body painting has blossomed around
the globe that is particularly popular among men. This is the practice of
painting the face with team colours at important sporting events. Bold,
graphic, often clever in design, these new experiments in body art have, at a
stroke, resurrected the peacock male – and in a context in which fears of
encroaching effeminacy are never entertained.

These dazzling faces that bejewel the stands at football matches also remind us that, however magnificent its artistic achievements, the cosmetic art of women in contemporary culture is almost always limited by a severe stylistic inhibition: namely, the need to respect and highlight the natural construction of the human face. Since antiquity, facial make-up in the West (and the same applies to 'higher' civilizations in the East) has served to adorn and emphasize the eyes, lips and contours of the face, the design always subservient to the physical shape. We find kohl or eyeliner employed to circle and delineate the eyes, lipstick to emphasize or modify the shape of the lips and graduated foundation shades to 'sculpt out' and enhance the cheekbones. This 'facial' style of make-up is found from ancient Egypt to this season's fashion catwalks, from Hollywood stars to the Japanese geisha. In the most extreme expression of this approach cosmetics are designed to completely disappear in the service of 'natural beauty'.

But when we look at body painting in tribal societies (or, indeed, in the contemporary example of sporting 'tribes') we see a very different approach in which colours, lines, swirls, dots and figurative motifs have been applied as if the physical features that they overlay are an irrelevance – the image is presented as if on an uninterrupted blank canvas. As Robert Brain puts it in *The Decorated Body* (within a discussion of Caduveo face painting in Brazil), such tribal peoples are happy to 'dislocate the face in the interests of their art...The natural harmony of the features is of less importance than the artificial harmony of the design. The Caduveo painter, asked to draw the design on a flat surface, draws not the face but the design, respecting its true proportions as if they were painted on a curved surface. To respect the face, she would have to distort the design, as in a Western photograph.' Presuming the greater importance of the design – a key symbolic focal point of her culture – the artist opts to distort the human face to the point at which it is unrecognizable to us. She does, in other words, what our approach to facial cosmetics almost always refuses to do.

We can, therefore, distinguish between two separate types of body or facial painting: one uses the human body as a canvas for the transmission of symbolic information and the other uses pigment and line to adjust and perfect the body itself. Tribal peoples – seeking to distance themselves from the natural world; passionately concerned with the expression of their culture – typically opted for

THE CONTEMPORARY PAINTED BODY has a world of different possibilities to choose from and embraces many cultures. *below* Fatima, born in the Netherlands, wears kohl eyeliner to emphasize her eyes and respects the traditions of her religion by wearing a headscarf; *opposite* American Karta wears face paint in a style reminiscent of tribal treatment of design, not emphasizing the features

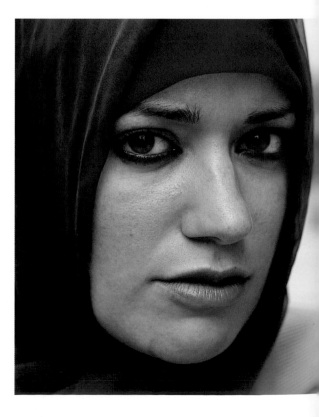

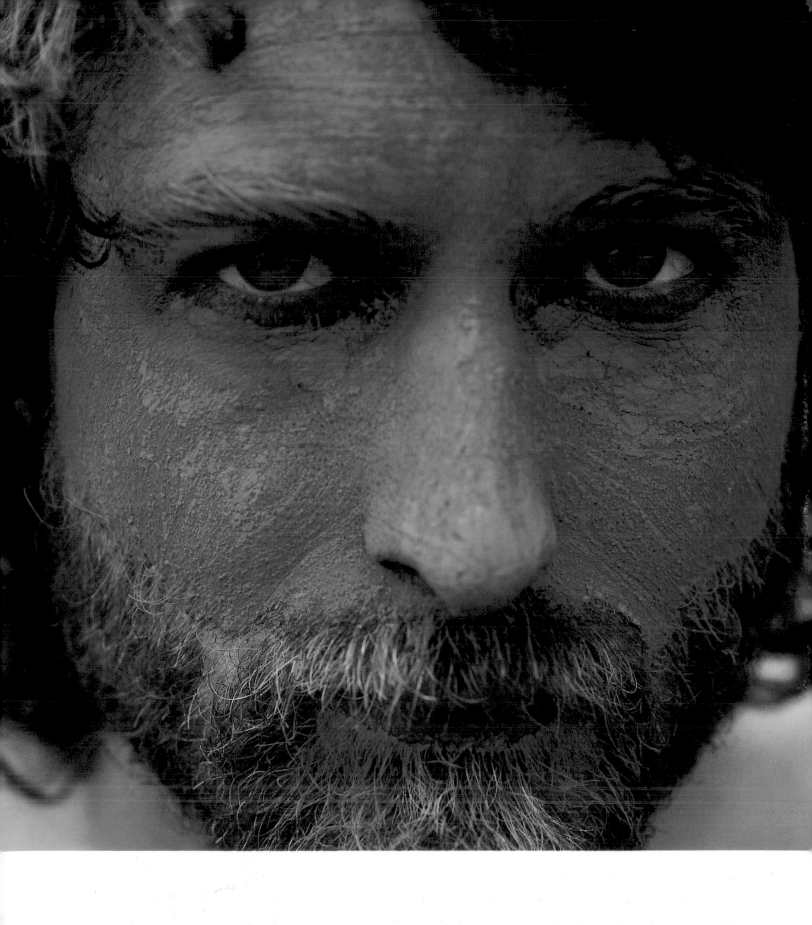

the primacy of message over medium. And the same is true of contemporary sports enthusiasts, their faces reduced to graphic adverts for their teams.

This distinction between informative and cosmetic approaches is useful in considering all of the various body art techniques. (Tattooing, for example, is typically highly informative, while plastic surgery is almost always purely cosmetic.) It is important, however, to appreciate that this distinction is only rarely absolute. Except in the specific instance of warpaint (where the goal is to look as horrible and frightening as possible), however informative a tribal person's body decoration, its effect is inevitably to make the body more beautiful. What says the right thing ('I am a member of this tribe'; 'I am in tune with the spirit world') also looks right. And no doubt the same principle holds true for the sports fan radiant in his or her team's colours.

On the other hand, even where cosmetics are used purely with the intention of rendering the face more beautiful, they inevitably seem to say something about the woman who wears them. This is because particular colours and styles of make-up have historical and personal associations that radiate with meaning. Whether it is intended or not, whether it is true or not, we infer very different personal information about a woman wearing black lipstick painted in sharp peaks than we do about a woman wearing pink, frosted lipstick applied following the lips' natural shape. If a pop star, the Queen or your friend Susan wears a particular shade of eyeshadow this will shape your presumptions about the next stranger you see who also happens to wear it. Unless it succeeds in actually disappearing from view, make-up never simply looks nice; it is always tinged with significance – even if, as is usually the case, it is hard to translate these messages in make-up consciously and literally. This shouldn't cause us to dismiss the significance of such visual communication. It is one of the underlying themes of this book that stylistic, non-verbal communication can often signify what verbal language cannot succeed in articulating and that this explains the continued importance of body decoration and dress as personal statement.

The cosmetic style of make-up (in which colour and line are at the service of the natural face) has proved amazingly entrenched in Western culture. The Mod girls of London in the early 1960s caused a stir with their white lipstick and enormous, painted-on eyelashes. The Psychedelics brought fluorescent shades into the make-up palette. The Punks and the Goths rendered the face skull-like

A UNISEX REVOLUTION
with make-up for men and lots of subcultural experimentation, predicted for decades in the media, has yet to materialize in the mainstream. Even a little eyeliner still has the power to challenge accepted notions of gender display. *opposite* Adam, a club DJ at Cyberdog and on the London hardcore techno scene, has a contemporary take on the Punk Mohican look, with shaven eyebrows and facial hair making his dark eye make-up all the more dramatic

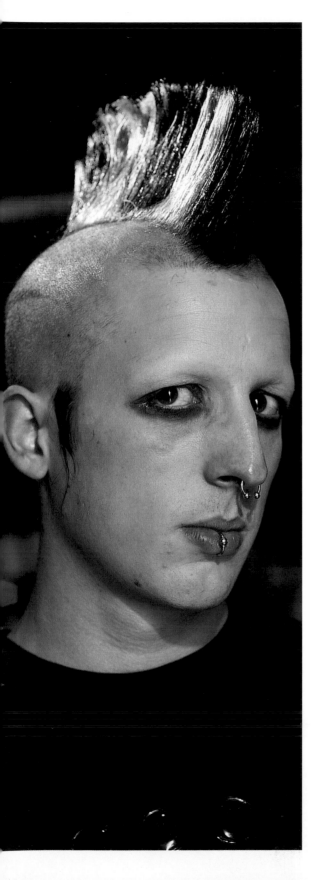

with abysmal eye sockets and pointy, macabre black lips. Yet in all these styles, and even in the case of Punk (despite its celebration of tribal influences in other respects) there was little in women's make-up that actually defied the traditional, cosmetic approach in which facial features are highlighted and shaped. One noteworthy exception was Jordan, the assistant at Vivienne Westwood and Malcolm McClaren's SEX shop on Carnaby Street who, for her starring role in Derek Jarman's film *Jubilee*, drew delicate but striking Cubist black lines across her entire face. A decade later, the influential and always experimental performance artist and professional dandy Leigh Bowery (once described by Boy George as 'an art work on two legs') regularly dispensed with all traditional make-up conventions by, for example, polka-dotting his face with colour or letting bright, molten wax drip down over his shaven head. No one else – let alone the masses – seems to have copied these great innovators.

Today, with make-up still by and large restricted to the role of adding colour and shape to the lips, the eyes and the cheekbones, it is a completely separate tradition of body painting, henna (or *mehndi*, as it is known in India), that offers the most exciting possibilities for resurfacing our skin with meaningful designs. Long developed as a body art in India, North Africa, the Middle East and Southeast Asia, this technique uses the ground leaves of the bright-green henna plant applied as a paste to the skin with the tip of a stick or a cone of paper or plastic (as if decorating a cake). Although ancient, natural henna body decoration became extremely popular in the late 1990s when worn by the likes of Madonna, Liv Tyler, Demi Moore, Prince and Naomi Campbell. While traditionally used to decorate only the hands and feet for important ritual occasions such as a wedding, we have discovered possibilities for using henna art on any part of the body and for daily use.

Longer lasting than most body painting (several weeks if correctly applied using strong henna), *mehndi* occupies a place between cosmetics and tattooing. This is appealing to those who want the commitment of a decoration that is not here today and gone tomorrow while avoiding the total permanence of a tattoo. Stylistically it provides a valued contrast to the cosmetic approach of make-up. For while *mehndi* is beautiful, it is also informative – an intricate, comprehensive system for inscribing the body with meaning. From each of its cultural roots, *mehndi* design compiles a dictionary of symbols. For example, within the Indian tradition a lotus flower denotes survival in challenging

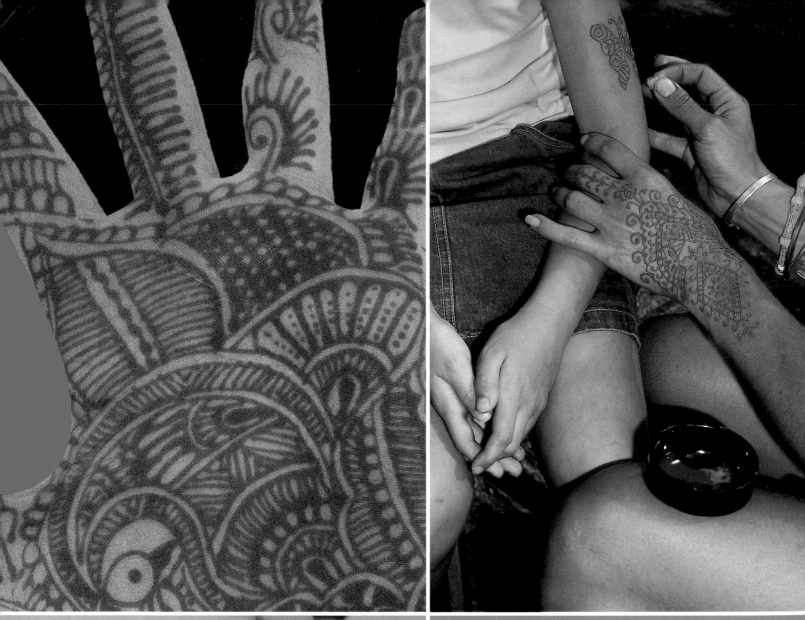

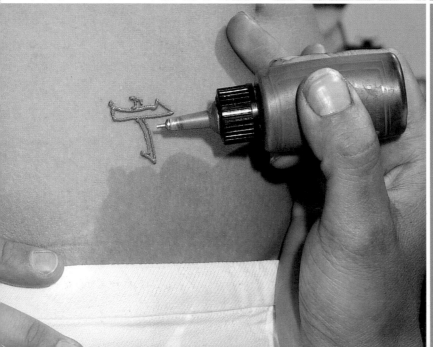

LONGER LASTING THAN MOST BODY PAINT,
henna (*mehndi*) is increasingly popular in the West.
Its long history in India, North Africa, the Middle East
and Southeast Asia and its associated symbolic and
aesthetic features (it is used to mark special occasions
and is traditionally applied to hands and feet) are part
of the appeal. Henna tattoo artists are often found
working on the street in summer. Use of artificial
(or 'black') henna can cause severe allergic reactions;
natural henna paste is green when applied. *This page*
and *opposite* henna designs by Danny, Netherlands,
who uses 'flash' books of her own designs; *left* Danny
applies a Chinese symbol of love to a teenage girl whose
friends also acquired symbolic henna tattoos as a ritual
to mark their friendship; *opposite* different stages in
the development of a henna tattoo, the left foot with
drying green henna paste, the right foot showing the
completed brownish-red tattoo

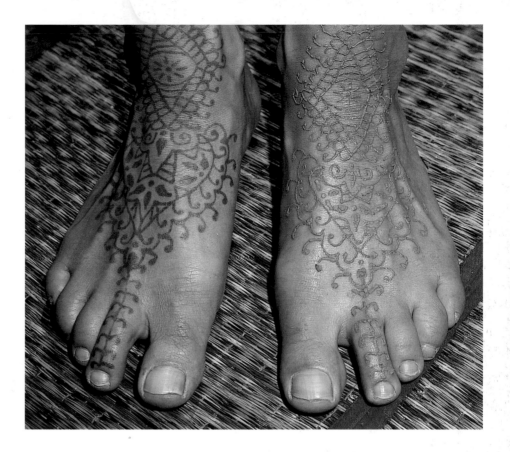

surroundings, the sun is 'the world door' (as Sumita Batra describes it in *The Art of Mehndi*) that opens onto knowledge and immortality, the peacock a symbol of love and desire, the swastika ('it is well') represents movement, happiness and good fortune. The art of henna as traditionally practised in North Africa, the Middle East and Southeast Asia operates according to different graphic rules, with different symbolic associations, but in all places it brings a spiritual and reflective significance to body art that Western make-up has rarely embraced. Meaningful and informative rather than simply cosmetic, traditional even within the context of its current trendiness, *mehndi* body art offers the opportunity for a return to the decorated body as intellectual and spiritual focus, a link with both the exotic and the ancient.

As well as painting designs or patches of colour onto our bodies, we humans have also often endeavoured to transform both the condition and the colour of our skin in its entirety. While Western women today (and, increasingly, men) often employ moisturizers to combat dry skin (and may be seen at the beach dripping suncreams and tanning oils) they generally do not want their skin to appear greasy – often using powder to give a matt rather than a shiny finish.

It is the opposite, however, among many traditional peoples. A woman of the Nuba of the Sudan would be so embarrassed to be seen without her body slicked with oil that, if none is available, she will hide indoors. Traditionally in parts of south-western Ghana, a young woman who is ready for marriage will have her body smeared liberally with shea butter before being paraded in front of prospective suitors. In societies such as these where vegetable oil or butter may be in short supply, these practices are probably explained by the symbolic association of greasiness with prosperity and well-being.

In Western society (and in the 'higher' cultures of the East), the symbolic association of light skin tone and high status has been more important. Tanning and darker skin colour is indicative of manual work outdoors, and so for hundreds of years powders and other lightening agents were employed to demonstrate aristocratic status. In his treatise *In Praise of Shadows*, the Japanese writer Junichirō Tanizaki speculates that the dark interiors of

A STATUS SYMBOL FOR CENTURIES
in both East and West, light skin was proof that someone was able to avoid outdoor labour. To highlight this effect, powders and paints were used throughout the world. *below* Tsjeggie, Belgium, shows off his suntan, fashionable in the West from the 1920s through association with expensive holidays and such sports as tennis; *opposite* Etsuko shows an interpretation of traditional Eastern style – in less dramatic form, lightened skin retains mainstream popularity in Japan

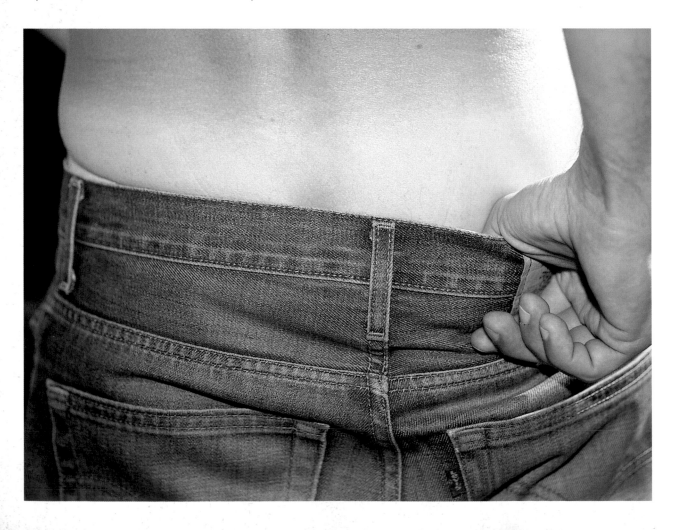

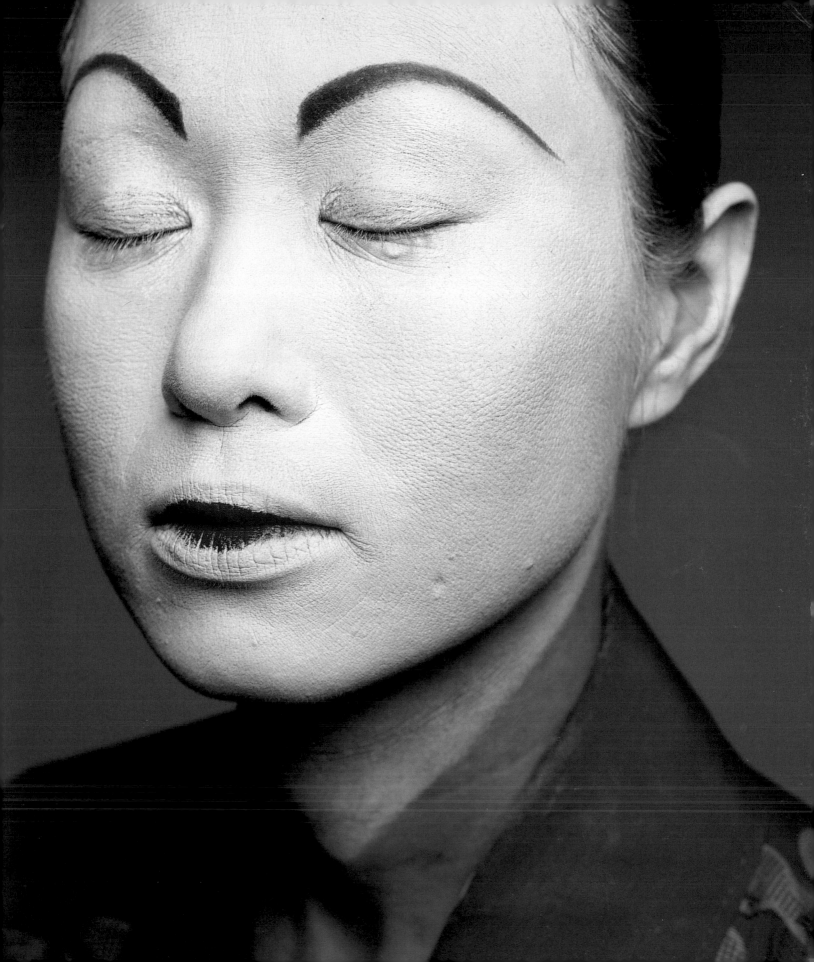

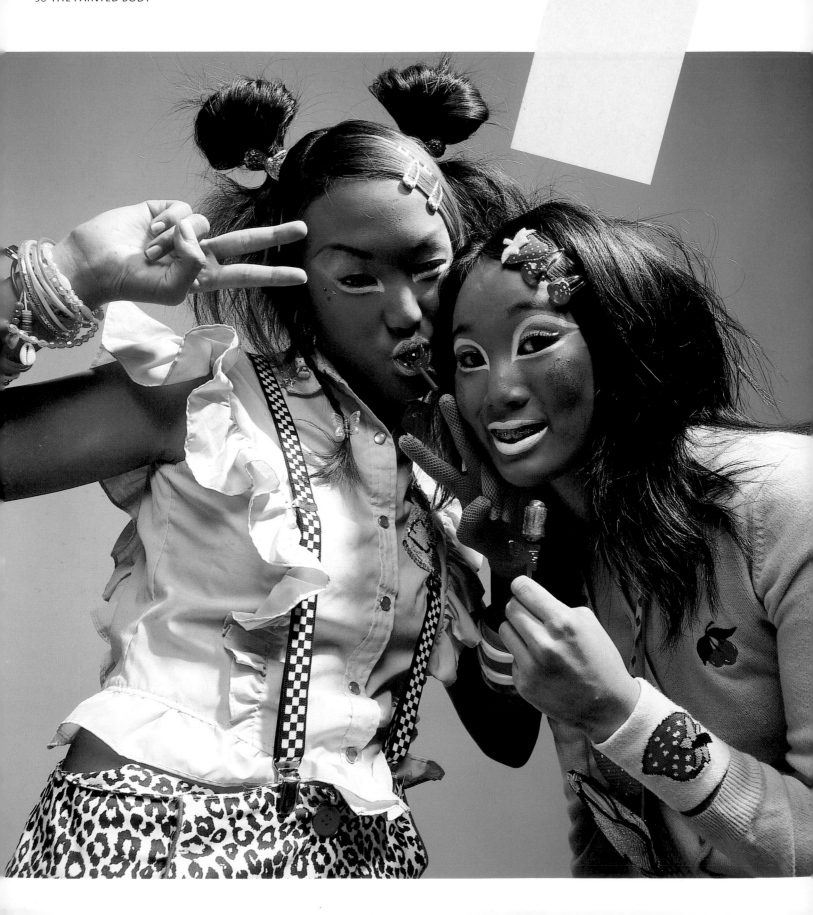

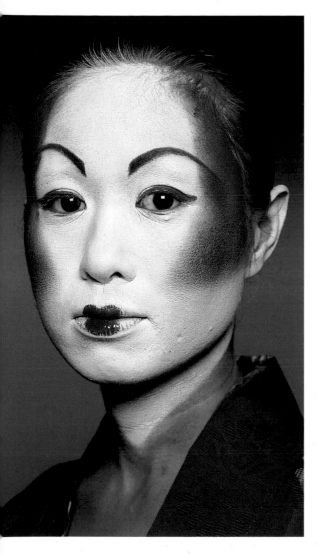

traditional Japanese buildings, the white face paints originally imported from China, the practice of blackening women's teeth and the classic, green, iridescent lipstick once favoured by Japanese women were all devised to highlight the 'supreme beauty' of women as 'the whitest of beings'.

This all changed in the West, however, in the 1920s when lazing in the sun on the French Riviera and participation in outdoor sports such as tennis reflected economic success and social status – with the result that the fashion designer Jean Patou invented the first suntan oil in 1927 and Ambre Solaire mass-produced its own product soon afterwards. This trend continued and intensified until the 1980s, when concerns about skin cancer and (probably of greater social importance) the wider availability of sea and sun (through package holidays) brought back the equation pale skin equals higher status, which equals beauty.

Yet in Japan (where full-page adverts for skin-lightening preparations are commonplace in glossy fashion magazines) one group of young women – the 'Black Face' Ganguro Girls – goes to great extremes to assert the beauty of very dark skin. Taking their inspiration from the heavily tanned skin of adult-video star turned TV celebrity Ai Iijima and the popularity of Hawaiian holidays, the Ganguro Girls devised a look that contrasted the darkest possible skin tones (usually achieved either on the sunbed or through the use of tanning lotions) with white lipstick, generously applied white eyeshadow and lightened hair tones. Highly distinctive, unique throughout the world in their revival of the heavily tanned look, the Ganguro Girls have played an interesting part in the remarkable emergence of Japan as the new wellspring of streetstyle creativity.

A CHALLENGE TO THE EQUATION
of beauty and high status with light skin, which persists in many parts of the East, Ganguro Girls delight in a heavily tanned appearance (often achieved on sunbeds), which is further accentuated with white lipstick and eyeshadow. *opposite* Joyce and Priscilla illustrate the Ganguro look; *above* Etsuko shows an interpretation of traditional Geisha make-up

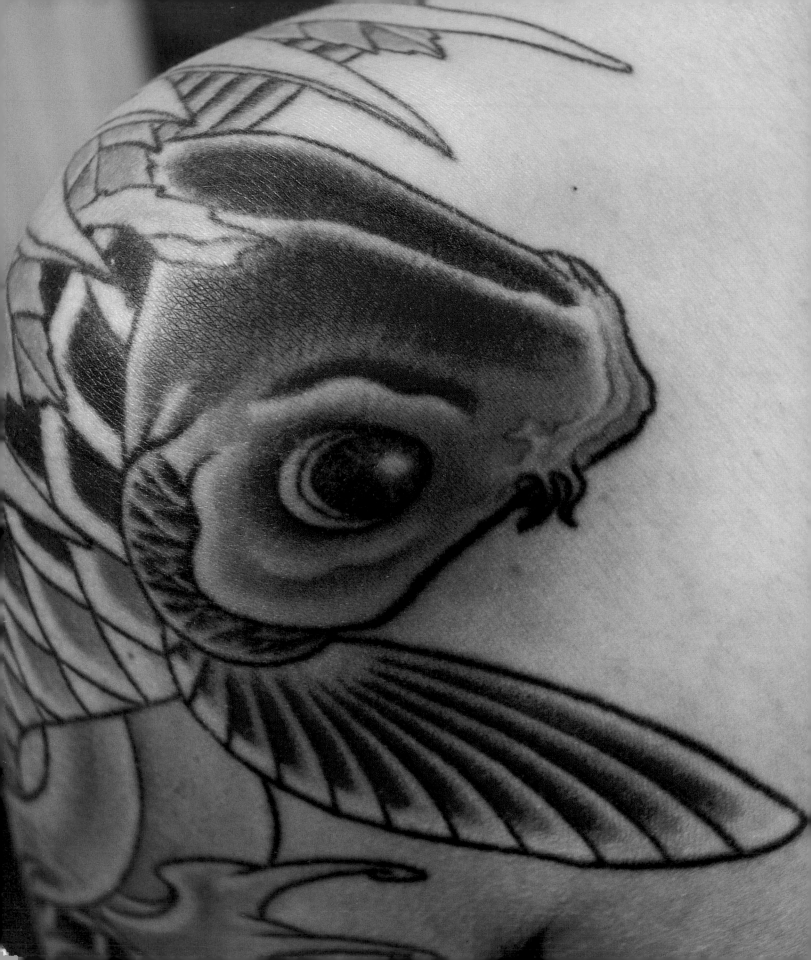

CHAPTER TWO

THE TATTOOED BODY

By putting colour into rather than on top of the skin, permanent markings can be created. Like body painting, this was probably also a chance discovery, the result of soot or clay getting into an open cut. Thorns or splinters of wood, bone, flint or shell could be used to puncture the skin to create deliberate permanent marks. More elaborately, a number of such sharp objects could be bound together and attached to a single wood or bone implement. Especially in the South Pacific, such clusters of sharp points were attached at a right angle to a stick, which could then be struck by another stick to drive the points into the skin. Distinctive tattooing technologies evolved among the Maori of New Zealand (their famous *moko* facial tattoos achieved by putting carbon pigment within scars chiselled into the flesh) and among Inuit populations where a needle and thread (smeared with soot) were drawn through the skin horizontal to the surface.

As in Japan and many other cultures, tattooing in the West was traditionally done with straight needles of varying thickness and configuration, which were prodded under the skin. Except for an ever-expanding palette of colours, the only significant development in tattoo technology came in 1891 when Samuel O'Reilly patented the first electric tattooing machine in New York. (As the early 20th-century British tattooist George Burchett points out in his autobiography, there is an interesting irony in the fact that 'Tattooing, the most ancient of all beauty treatments, was the very first to make use of electricity.')

CONTEMPORARY TATTOO DESIGN
in classic Japanese style. *these pages* Lina, Sweden, shoulder tattoo by Rob Admiraal

But long before O'Reilly's 'tattaugraph', an extremely wide range of cultures throughout the world – from the Ukraine to Japan, Alaska to the South Pacific – had developed extraordinarily complex and graphically striking tattoo styles. The range, grace and complexity of so many of these styles obliges us to accord tattoo-ing the status of one of humankind's most sophisticated artistic genres. That this art form uses the living human body as its canvas underlines rather than detracts from its aesthetic accomplishments – for this is a genre that offers scant latitude for mistakes. How many of our great masterpieces of 'fine art' required the rethinking and adjustment that are unavailable to the tattoo artist?

As well as a formidable aesthetic achievement, the tattooed body demands respect as a system of communication. Arguably the most informative of all forms of body art, the symbolic functions of tattooing are particularly impor-tant in societies that lack written language – its images, pictographs, abstract design motifs, colours and positioning on the body (itself a primal symbol: the 'social body') providing a crucial databank of the knowledge, beliefs, values and history of so many traditional cultures. Additionally, the contrasting tattoo styles of particular individuals within a group often articulate and underline differences in role and status – immediately identifying the chief, those who have shown courage in battle or prowess in the hunt as well as who is (and who is not) a fully fledged adult member of the tribe.

Possessing written language does not, however, eradicate the significance of tattoo design as a valuable medium of expression. Many modern 'tribes' – Bikers, Skinheads, Punks, Mexican-American Chicanos and countless street gangs – have used tattoos both to mark the members of their group and also to articulate the world view of their subculture symbolically. However, in today's world, it is the language of personal, individual identity – rather than the lan-guage of social commitment and shared values – that the tattoo is most often called upon to express.

Permanent and often painful, the tattoo introduces a more radical approach to transforming appearance than those previously discussed. Western society went through a long period of resistance to all such permanent decorations but in recent times this very quality, this challenge to transience, has con-tributed to the ever-growing appeal of both tattooing and body piercing.

In much the same way, the pain and bloodletting inherent in the tattooing process – once seen as the crucial proof of its barbarism – has also recently

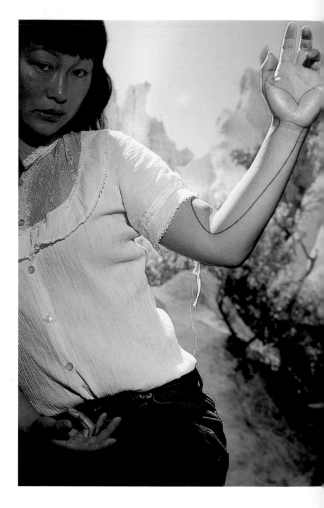

A NEW BREED OF TATTOO CUSTOMERS
demands ever more innovative, original designs from a new breed of tattooists scouring the world for inspiration. Although tattooing has an ancient history in the West, a broader group of enthusiasts and wider range of design styles has increased its popularity in recent decades. *above* Sun designed the fish tattoo on her arm and flower on her finger, executed by Rob Admiraal: 'Fish are beautiful animals but really my tattoos are abstract'; *opposite from top left, clockwise* Cecilia, skull tattoo on shoulder by Rob Admiraal; Anthony, a hairdresser at Lemonhead, with Japanese and Tribal torso tats; Caroline, North Star tattoos on her wrists; Lina, black panther tattoo by Mark; Marianne, an architect of 60, has her wrist tattoo as 'a permanent reminder of my deceased husband, the love of my life'; Peter got his tattoo with three friends, as a ritual – a visualization of the Dutch saying 'a little house, a little tree, a little pet', which encompasses the concept of settling down, a transition into adulthood (though the design omits the pet, a hint at rebellion). 'Stars and Flames', a full sleeve tattoo design by Michelle Myles at Dare Devil Tattoo. This design was inked onto a New York chef, Chris Santos.

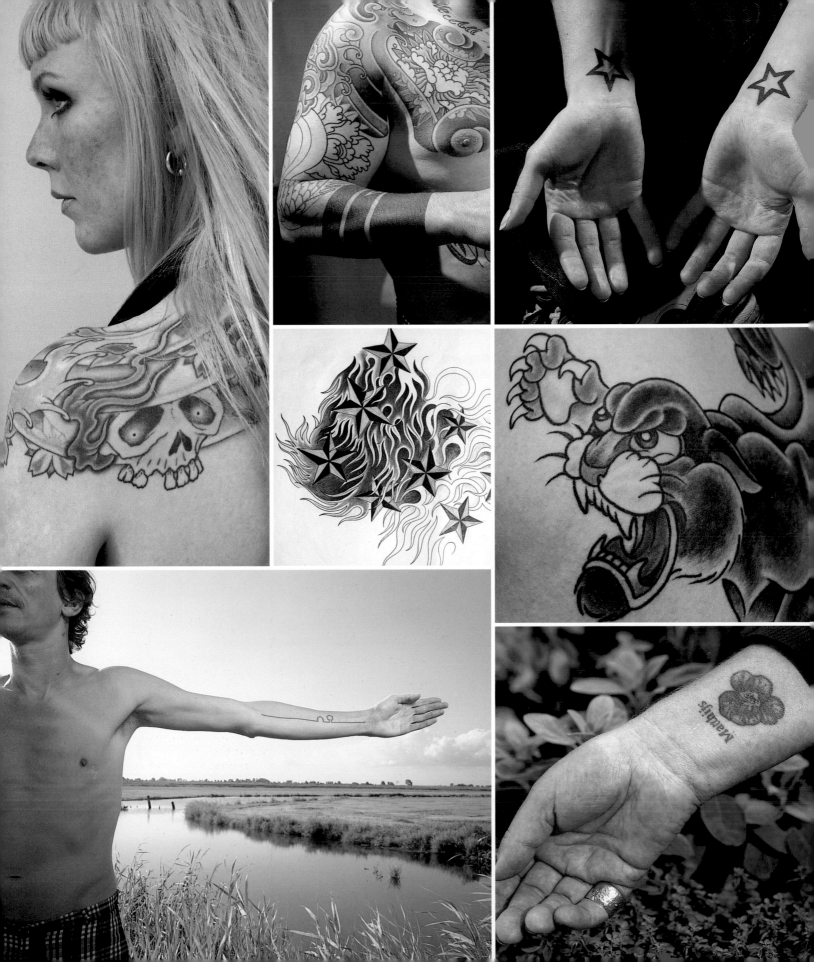

become, for many, part of this adornment's appeal: an act that demands such a level of commitment and courage being seen as uniquely valuable in a world where value has arguably lost all meaning except that of price.

When Captain James Cook 'discovered' Polynesia for the British in 1769, from a Western perspective he appeared to have discovered tattooing as well. Indeed, the English word for this technique of body decoration (and that of most European languages) derives from the Tahitian word *tatu* or *tatau* (to mark or strike the skin), which mimics the sound of one stick striking another to puncture the skin – the Tahitian technique of tattooing. Ironically, however, Europe has as much if not more historical claim to the invention of tattooing as does Polynesia. Perhaps people in the West in the 18th century had long forgotten the original meaning of previously used European terms for tattooing such as 'listing', 'rasing', 'pricking', 'pinking' and 'pouncing'. Perhaps they had come to associate the older term 'stigma' (Latin, from Greek for 'marks on the skin', from *stig-*, the stem of *stizein*, 'to prick') only with the marks on Christ's hands and feet (the plural, stigmata). Or perhaps, especially in the 18th-century Britain of Captain Cook, it was simply culturally convenient to forget such things. For once upon a time the shoe had been on the other foot: when the Romans 'discovered' Britain they called its inhabitants 'Picts' or 'painted people' because their bodies were covered in either body paint or, more likely, tattoos.

At any rate, from the 18th century onwards, for Europeans tattooing became inexorably linked with the exotic – something that strange peoples in very distant lands did to their bodies. Westerners became fascinated by this remarkable phenomenon and paid to see exhibitions of imported tribal peoples and tattooed European men who claimed to have been kidnapped and forcibly decorated at the hands of barbarians. (A fascinating myth, but one that fails to understand that traditional peoples permit only those they honour to be tattooed.) Many who travelled to the Pacific – some explorers, and many sailors of all ranks – delighted in the tattoos that they acquired there. In later centuries, after Japan had been opened to the world in 1854 and the artistry of its tattoo masters celebrated abroad (while, ironically, outlawed at home for the Japanese themselves), many made the journey – most famously George V of Britain and Tsar Nicholas II of Russia – specifically to acquire such distinctive, exotic and beautiful decorations.

A REDISCOVERY AND REVIVAL

of classic, heart-felt tats has recently taken place. Traditional Western tattoo styles, which fell out of favour during the tattoo renaissance when exotic styles were introduced, are enjoying new popularity and interpretation. *below* Daan wears a transfer tattoo from inside a bubblegum packet; *below right* Tea describes her arm tatto by Rhonda Hulzen as 'a dyke wink to sailors' tattoos of sexy pin-ups'

Another such Westerner was the aforementioned George Burchett, who applied the knowledge he acquired as a seaman in Asia to his work as a tattooist in London from 1900 to 1953. The American tattooist Gus Wagner was a seaman in the Pacific during the same period and when he set up his own tattoo parlour in Newark, Ohio, he brought knowledge (and even tools) he had acquired in Borneo and Java.

Burchett, Wagner and many others brought a skill and imagination to their profession that produced many beautiful tattoos, but, in the main, tattooing as practised in Britain, Europe and America degenerated aesthetically to become hackneyed, two-dimensional, often crude and repetitive. Most customers were

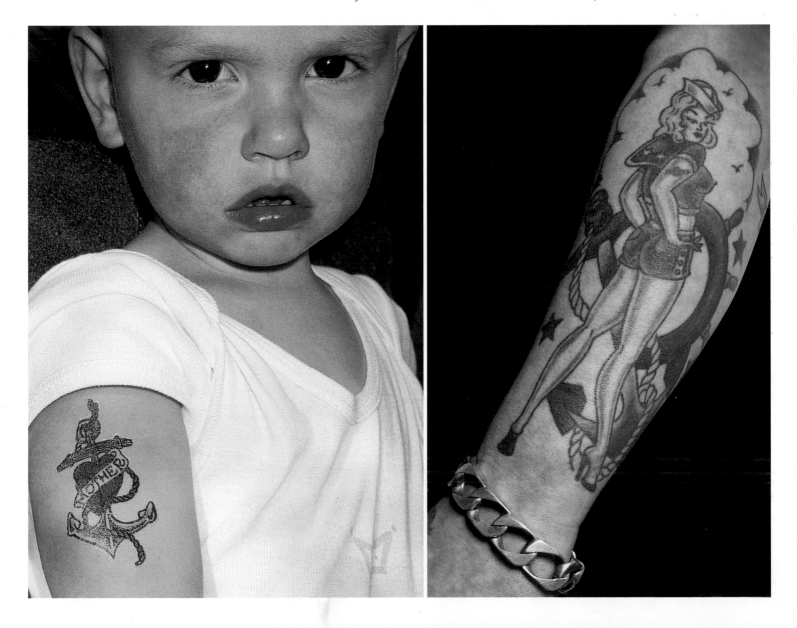

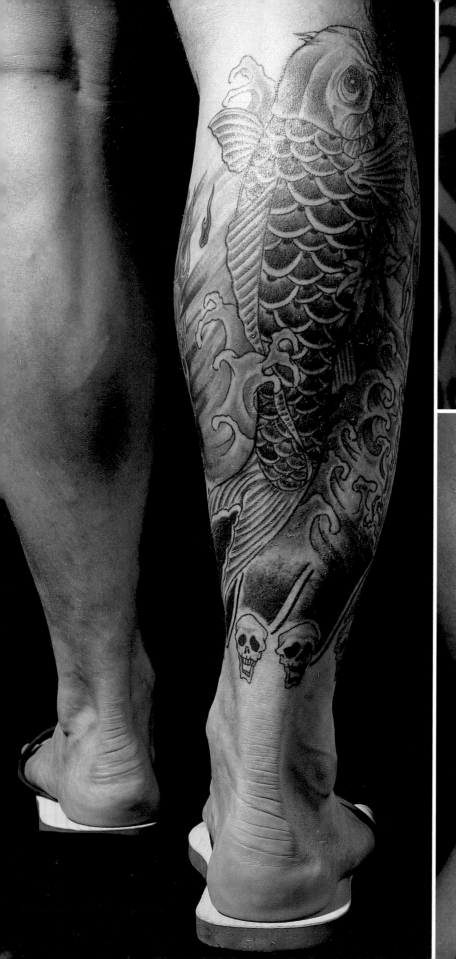
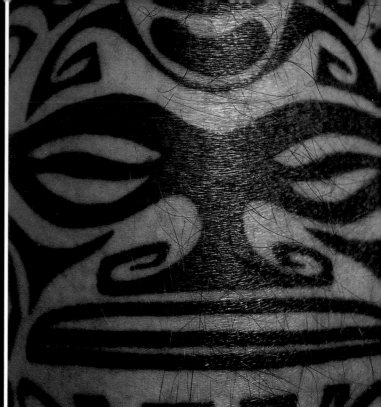
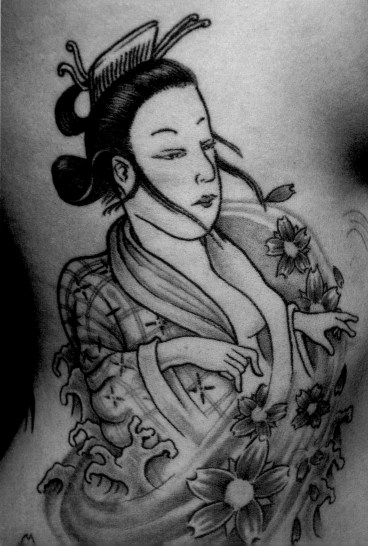

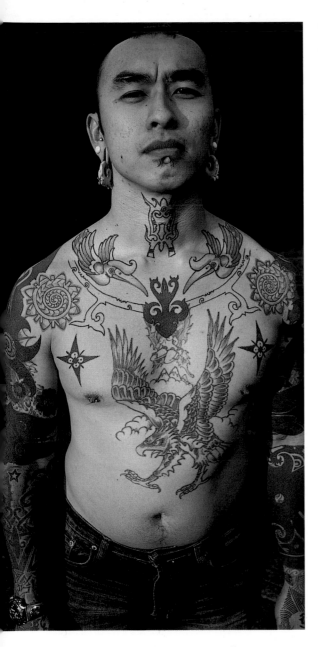

forced to choose from a standard set of near-identical 'flash' drawings found on the walls of studios from Hamburg to San Francisco, which were simply stencilled onto the skin with little or no sensitivity to placement on the body. Writing in 1953, in *Pierced Hearts and True Love* (one of the first general histories of tattooing), Hanns Ebensten describes such European and American tattoos as 'haphazard', 'hurriedly drawn and badly executed', 'spaced without thought or deliberation' and placed 'in an unpleasant relationship to each other'.

Unfortunately, while there are some noteworthy exceptions, Ebensten was right about the standards of Western tattooing at that time. But while the general view is that blame for this aesthetic failure rests on artistically inept and money-hungry tattooists (of which, no doubt, there were many), it is more rewarding to consider how features of the Western world view made it next to impossible for even the most talented and dedicated European or American tattooist to equal or surpass the art of Japan or the technologically simpler societies of the Pacific. (Or that of the Scythians of the Ukraine some two thousand years ago: the body of a Scythian chief found preserved in permafrost possesses exquisite tattoos of real and imaginary animals positioned with breathtaking grace around his body.)

Unlike the Scythians, the Pacific Islanders, the Japanese and so many others, Westerners in their tattooing had not come to terms with the human body as a unique, three-dimensional object. Inevitably, this failure forces us to consider the West's problematic relationship with the human body itself. In the traditional Western view, the flesh is weak, it leads us astray, it debilitates and limits us and, most importantly, it is alien, extraneous, not us. (This peculiar attitude begins with Plato but was formalized by Descartes' famous dictum, which divides between physical and mental experience and equates being with the latter, ignoring the significance of the former.) Given such cultural baggage, is it any wonder that until recent times Western tattooists found it so difficult to approach the medium of the human body with the respect and delight that is so evident in other tattoo traditions?

Whereas the Japanese or Tahitian tattooist had always worked with the body, the traditional Western tattooist seemed determined to cover it with art — in the process treating the three-dimensional body as if it were nothing but a two-dimensional blank sheet of paper. And if it didn't occur to him to use a consistent background to join together separate images into a visual whole (as the

A WIDE RANGE OF PACIFIC TATTOO STYLES is recognized internationally as accomplished aesthetic achievement. The tattoo renaissance learned in particular from Borneo, Polynesia, Micronesia and Japan. *opposite from far left, clockwise* Nick, UK, legpiece: 'I developed the design from the famous woodcut of a wave by Hokusai. The elements fire and water feature strongly and the seven skulls represent the seven deadly sins'; Henni, Tahitian-style leg piece; Jannetje, Geisha girl, all by Giorgio at Fox Tattoo; *above* Marc, tattoos inspired by and collected during his travels in Borneo and Australia, by a range of artists

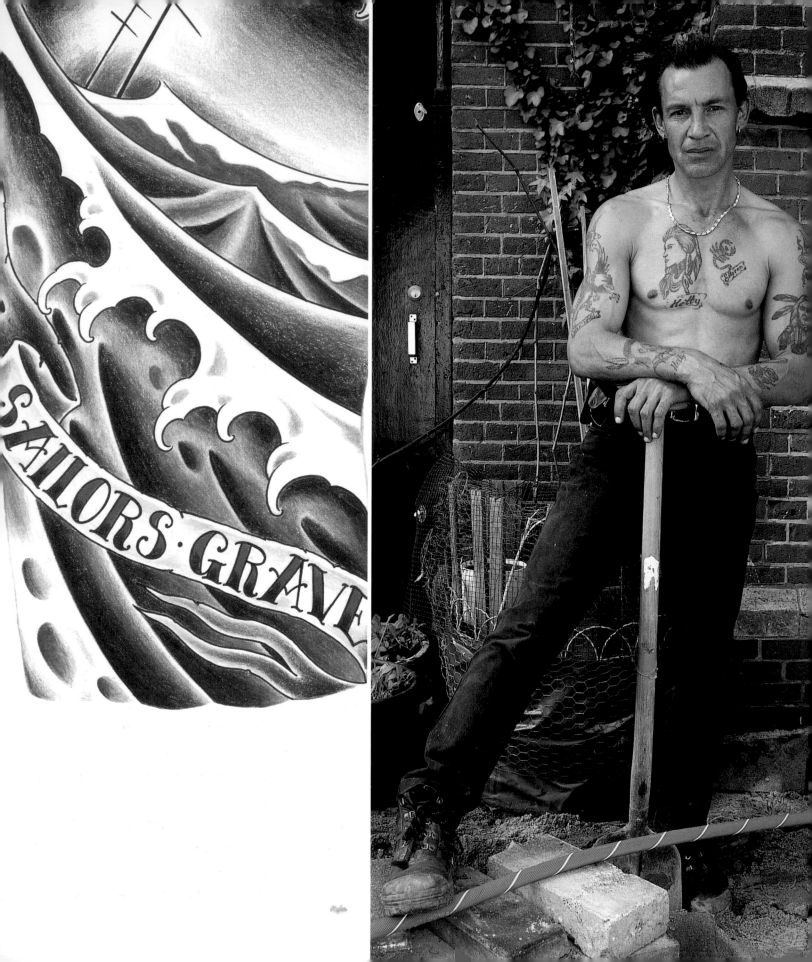

Japanese do), this is because, in the Western tattoo tradition, each image was executed as if on its own, separate, flat plane. (There is an interesting contrast here with Western cosmetic art, which, as discussed in the previous chapter of this book, almost always enhances, respects and celebrates the natural contours of the face. The key difference is gender. As Western men became increasingly estranged from their own bodies Western women were increasingly obliged to equate self with physicality. It should come as no surprise, therefore, that tattooing – a form of body decoration that existed in the West as an almost uniquely masculine adornment – should neglect the physical medium of the body in favour of the message inscribed on it, whereas cosmetics for women made and still make the medium of the face the message.)

If the traditional Western tattooist was limited by his lack of respect for the human body, he also suffered from too much respect for the art world (which in the West, perhaps uniquely, had come to exclude body art from its domain). Striving to assert their own and their profession's artistic credentials, Western tattooists delighted in etching studies of 'great' paintings onto their clients' backs and chests. And even when an image had no such fine art parentage, it was invariably drawn onto the skin in a painterly style. This persistence in trying to ape fine art inhibited Western tattooing from developing its own style – one more suited to its own tools and medium. It also kept tattoo art resolutely figurative: even when Western fine art discovered the possibilities of abstraction in the 1920s tattoos failed to follow suit.

Until, that is, the 1960s – when a new generation of tattooists kick-started the 'tattoo renaissance'. As some of the fledging tattooists (for example, Cliff Raven and Ed Hardy) had been to art college in the 1950s and early 1960s, they brought with them a broader, 20th-century vision of what art could be – even embracing non-figurative styles such as abstraction. Alternatively, as in the case of the great pioneer of the tattoo renaissance 'Sailor Jerry' Collins, increased awareness of the aesthetic possibilities of tattoo art came from direct contact with tattooing in the Pacific. As discussed earlier, this was hardly the first time Western tattooists had directly experienced Eastern tattooing, but in the 1950s changing perceptions of both other cultures and the nature of art – together with a more positive view of the human body – meant that the likes of Collins and his followers could see the tattoo art of other peoples with fresh eyes.

A REAPPRAISAL OF 'FOLK STYLE'
has brought new respect to the Western tattoo tradition and inspiration to tattoo artists. No longer overshadowed by enthusiasm for exotic designs, the roots and designs of tattoos favoured by, for example, Western sailors, are explored afresh. *opposite left* tattoo design by Alex Binnie, drawing inspiration from imagery of sailors' tattoos combined with a wave pattern in the Japanese style; *opposite* Jeroen, a road digger with traditional Western tattoos placed discretely on the body

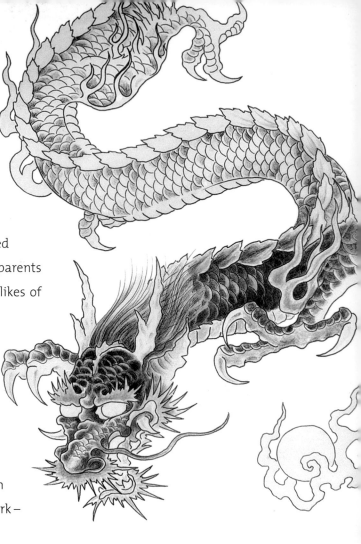

The tattoo renaissance may well have remained confined to the experiments of a handful of enthusiasts were it not for the youthquake and counterculture revolutions that shook the world in the second half of the 1960s. As well as a general questioning of mainstream cultural values and an accreditation of working/lower-class styles, this systemic shift also, for many, recast the criminal outlaw as folk hero. All of these strands of rebellion pointed towards a more positive view of tattooing. If we were the people our parents warned us about then we really should get some tattoos. When the likes of Janis Joplin, Joan Baez and Peter Fonda got their 'tats' it finally opened the floodgates once and for all. As with the counterculture itself, a significant proportion of these new tattoo enthusiasts were middle-class and college or art-school educated.

This juxtaposition of a new type of tattooist and a new type of customer brought about a creative explosion that shattered the mould of traditional Western tattooing. Instead of making a quick (perhaps inebriated) choice of design from hackneyed, standardized flash drawings, the customer was now more likely to want unique, custom work – developed through a creative collaboration between client and tattooist.

Ancient styles from other, exotic tattoo traditions (Tribal, Japanese, Celtic) now joined with new approaches coming from Modern Art (a Kandinsky or Miró etched on human flesh), influences from streetstyle and pop culture to expand the tattoo lexicon dramatically. For the first time we see Western designs that are positioned to respect and complement the three-dimensional shape of the human body. True to the spirit of Postmodernism, eclectic stylistic elements from around the world and from different historical periods were merged on one body or even within one tattoo. The colour palette widened yet further and adventurous experiments in finding new tools and modifying old ones bore fruit. Hygiene standards were raised: needles and other equipment were scrupulously sterilized in autoclaves and leftover inks thrown away rather than shared between separate customers.

In another important demographic shift, female customers (and, increasingly, female professional tattooists) have become commonplace. While the West has long had tattooed women, they were previously seen as so freakish and unusual as to be exhibited in circus sideshows and the like.

INTEGRATING SEPARATE ELEMENTS
into a visual whole, designing with respect for the shape of the body – Pacific tattoo traditions are now influencing Western design (which traditionally treated the body as a flat surface, designs bearing no aesthetic relationship to each other like graffiti scribbled on a wall at different times by different artists). *above* 'Red dragon' sleeve design by Michelle Myles at Dare Devil Tattoo, showing Japanese influence, later tattooed on a dancer; *opposite* Marco, tattoo in a continuous design

AN ADVERTISEMENT OF PERSONAL IDENTITY,
more and more people today create a distinctive, unique appearance style to escape the conformity of global culture. Such presentations of self increasingly include self-designed tattoos. *overleaf left* Sun, Korea, line drawing of a tree on shoulder: 'You can interpret my tattoos in your own way'; *overleaf right* Sharon, Netherlands, with tattoo mixing Celtic and Pacific styles under her pinstripe skirt and shirt

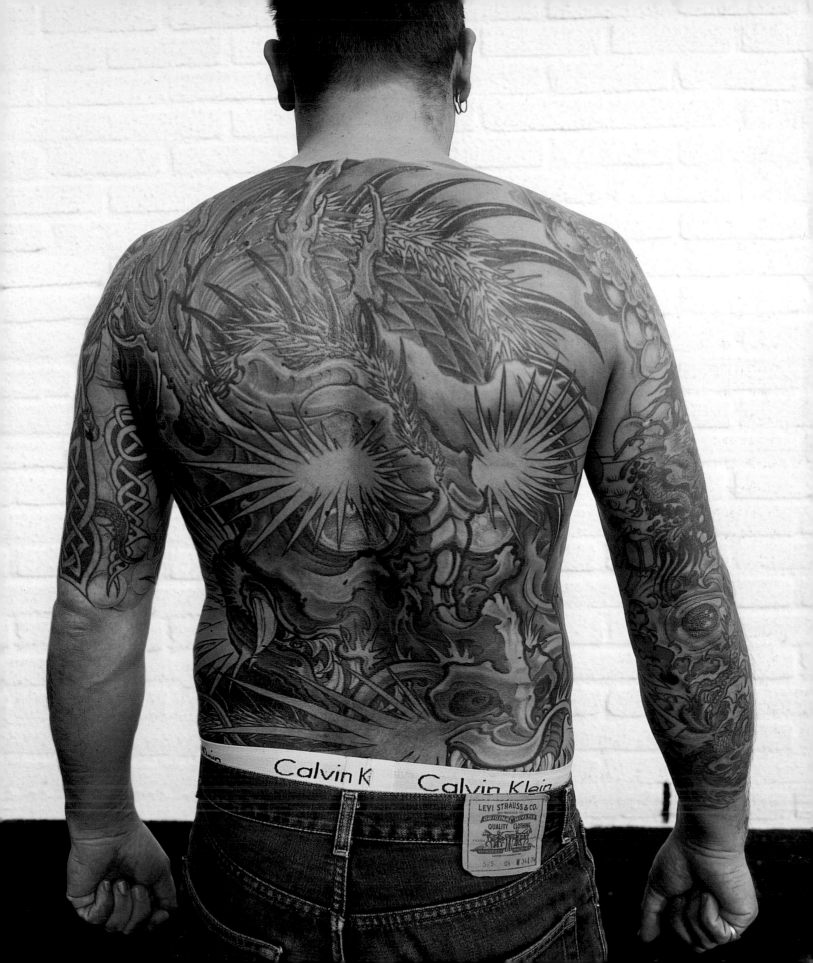

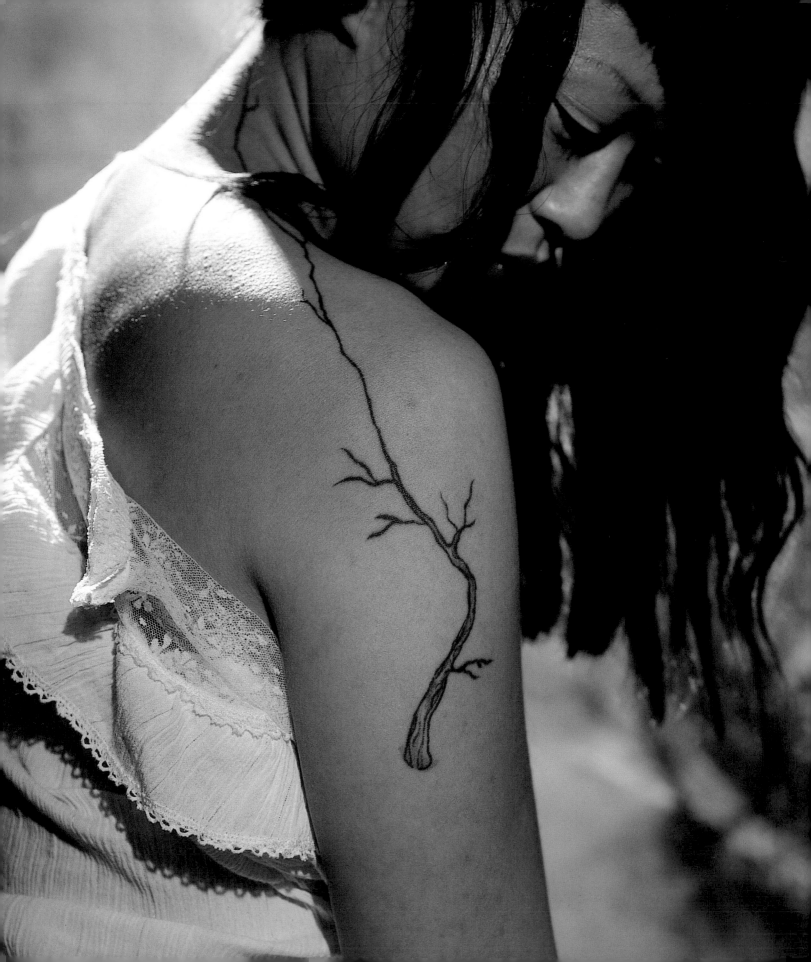

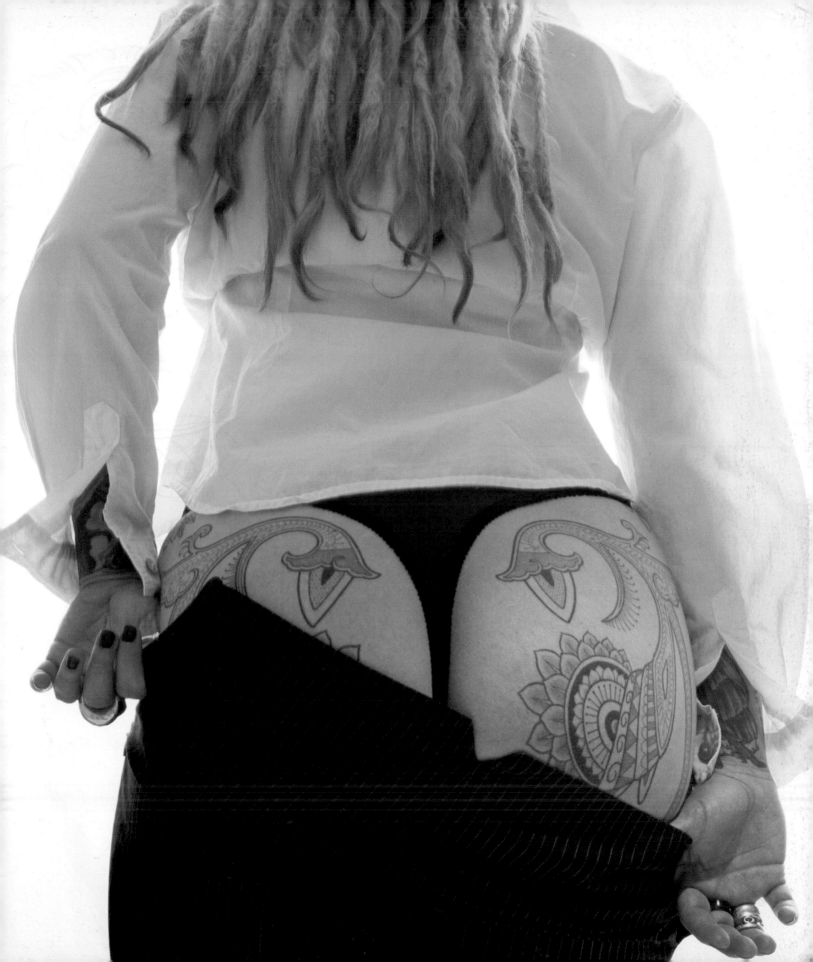

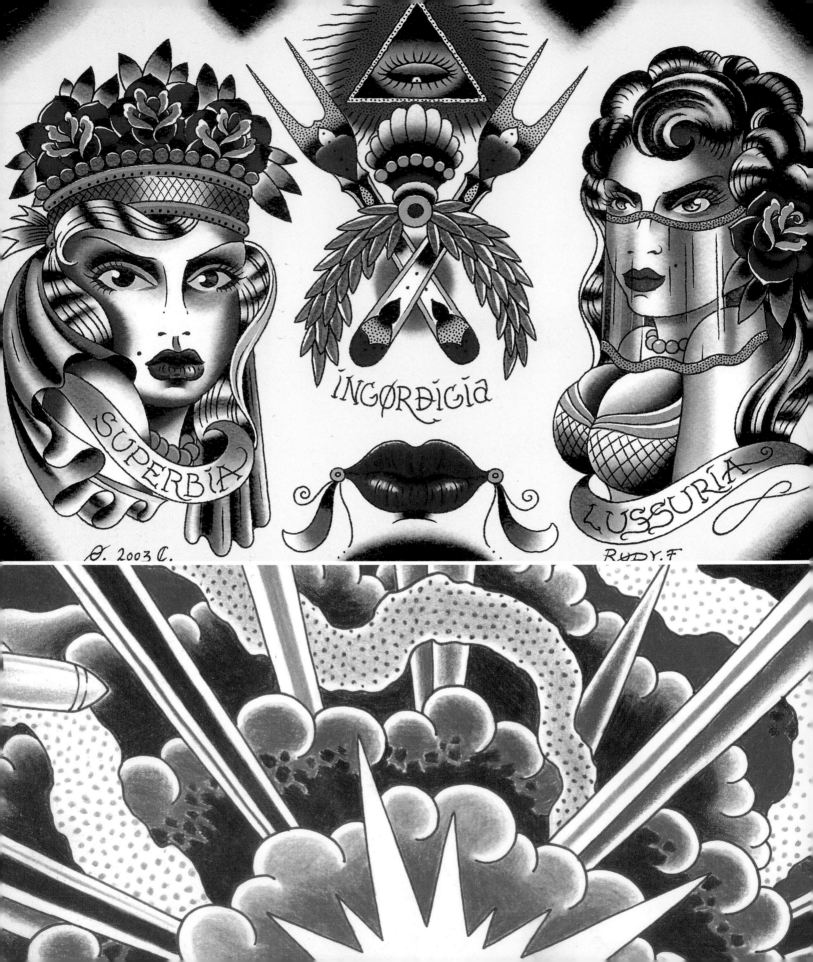

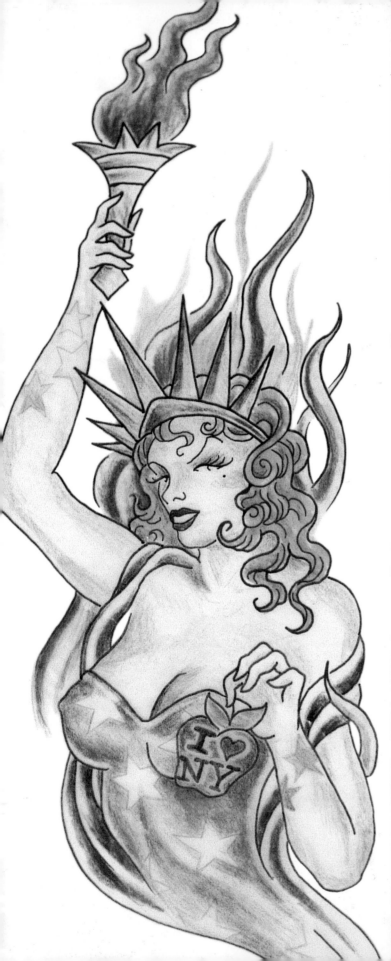

ABSORBING AESTHETIC INFLUENCES
from around the world and throughout history, but
fusing or reinterpreting them in unexpected ways,
tattoo artists today are creating dynamic new tattoo
styles. *opposite above* 'Pride, Greed and Lust' from
'Seven Deadly Sins' series by Rudy Fritsch at Original
Classic Tattoo; *opposite below* 'Bomb' by Alex Binnie
at Into You; *left* this 'Saucy Statue of Liberty' by
Michelle Myles at Dare Devil Tattoo took on new
significance during its design in September 2001
when NYC was attacked; *below* 'Snake Lady' by
Amanda Toy at Original Classic Tattoo mixes
manga, voodoo and traditional influences

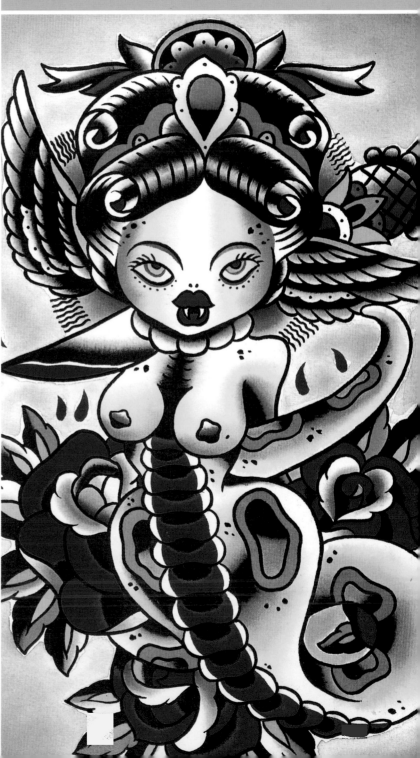

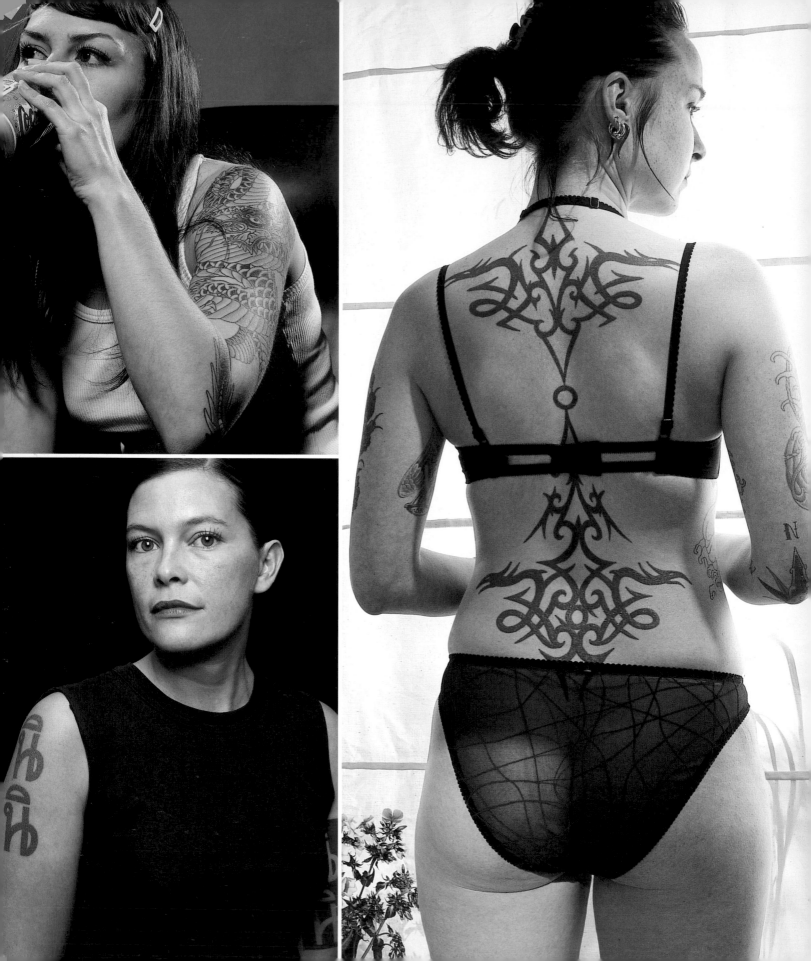

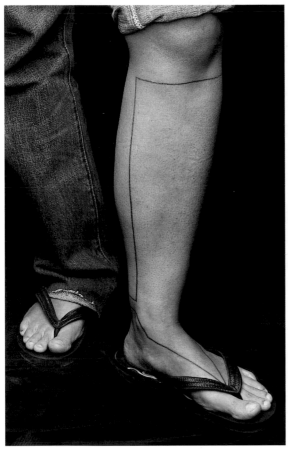

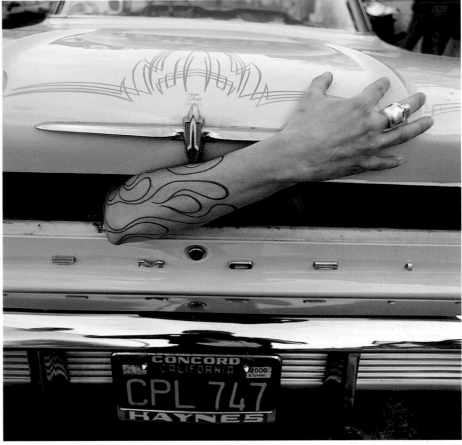

INSPIRATION FOR A TATTOO

is as individual as its design and placement on the body, whether it comes from an exotic culture, an emotional journey or a lifestyle. Original ideas are developed in collaboration with a tattoo artist, creating a tattoo signalling the values of the customer. *opposite top left* Caroline, Japanese-style dragon sleeve by Rob Admiraal; *opposite* Jannetje, Celtic-influenced back-piece by Sjap at House of Tattoos; *opposite bottom left* Margit, 'It took me 15 years of thinking what kind of design I would like to have. After a trip to Thailand with my friend Vanessa (subsequently the designer of all my tattoos) I had the idea to put my sister's name on my arm; she died in May 1981. The first one was put on my right arm in 2000. That year I had a lot of pain in the left side of my body; a year later I put the second tattoo on my left arm. Two months later the doctors noticed a tumour. After three operations, I wanted a third tattoo to end this horrible time – a shield, to protect me for the rest of my life!' *seen above* outlined on Margit's leg; *above right* Dean, flame tattoo inspired by Von Dutch, 1950s Hot Rod pinstriper

Only a generation ago, tattooing (presumably because of the pain involved) constituted one, unique form of body adornment that didn't call into question a 'real' man's masculinity. But now, directly paralleling what has happened in clothing (it is difficult to find a woman today who doesn't wear jeans or trousers, but a man in a skirt or dress is still seen as a transvestite), the old masculine fortress of tattooing has been successfully stormed by the female sex.

All these factors combined have made tattooing one of the most exciting and imaginative contemporary art forms. As can be seen at any of the growing number of tattoo conventions or on the pages of the many magazines and websites devoted to this body art, hundreds of thousands, if not millions of people are now actively engaged in stretching the aesthetic and stylistic possibilities of the tattoo.

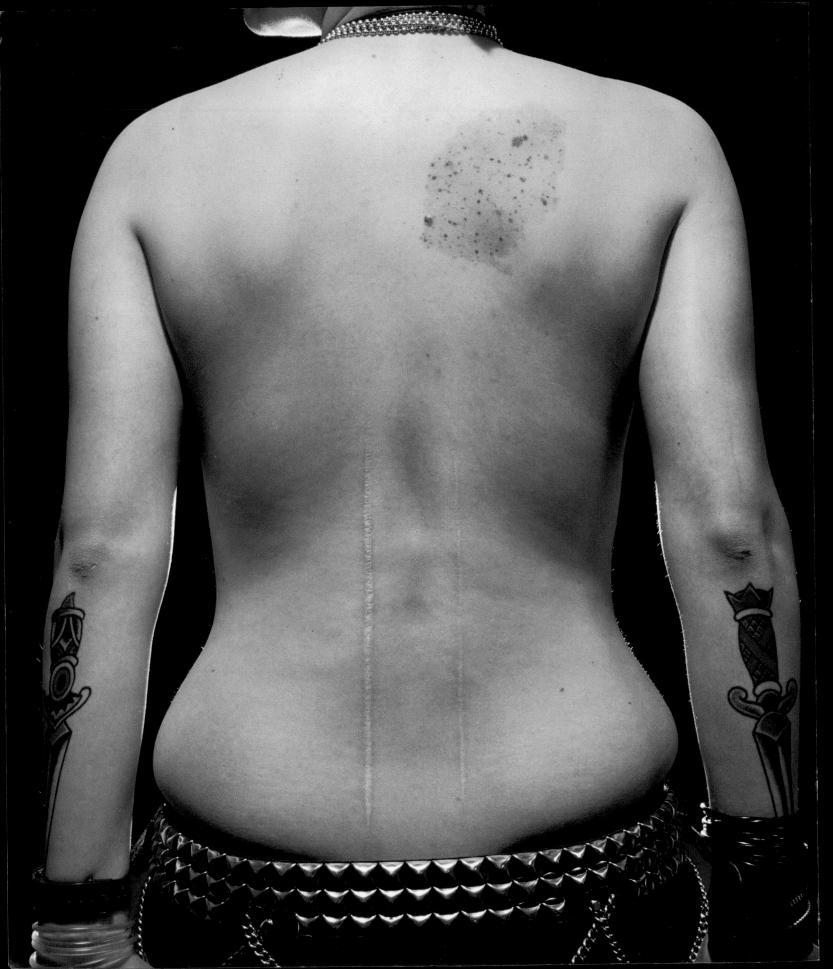

CHAPTER THREE

THE SCARRED BODY

The idea of deliberately cutting decorative patterns into the skin seems particularly barbaric to most people in contemporary society. Aside from the all too obvious pain, there is the high level of bloodletting involved. Compared with tattooing, which can achieve great subtlety and intricacy in its design, the results of scarification – at least to Western eyes – seem aesthetically limited. Finally, with little if any history of this form of body decoration within Western cultural tradition, scarification seems especially alien and 'primitive'. (In fact, among German students there was a tradition of deliberately inflicting fencing scars until the 20th century; but the haphazardness of such marks limited their artistic merit.)

In contrast, and probably because tattooing is less effective on black skin, scarification has a long history throughout Africa, where an extremely wide range of cultures saw it as an essential aspect of beauty – a tactile as well as visual feature of any attractive, desirable body. Given that Africa is now widely recognized as the homeland of our species, and that scarification has been found so extensively throughout this continent, it is not unreasonable to see the deliberately scarred body as an extremely ancient feature of human life – the body art technique first used by our most distant ancestors to set themselves apart from all other animals permanently and irrefutably; the art that most immediately and profoundly made visible our species' cultural distancing from nature; and all the while, the scarred body and the beautiful body becoming increasingly synonymous.

AN UNUSUAL AND DISTINCTIVE
permanent body decoration. *these pages* Anja, Finland, scarification created using fish hooks

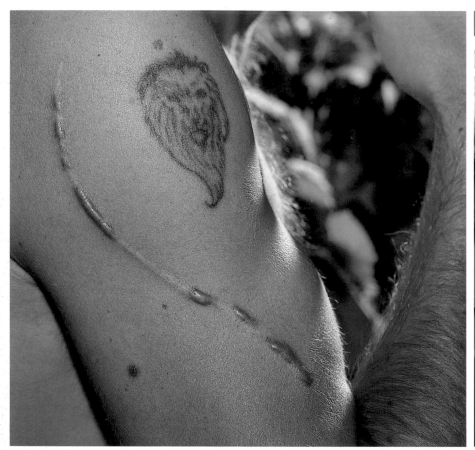

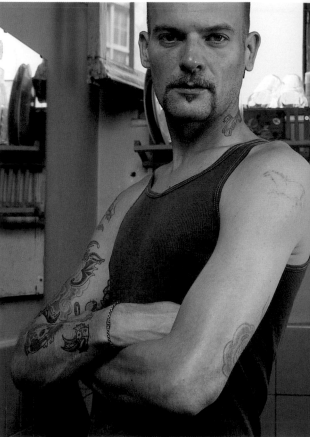

The implements used and the preferred styles of scarification varied considerably from region to region, culture to culture, but the technique was essentially the same: a sharp piece of flint, bone, shell, bamboo (or, in more recent times, a metal nail, knife or razor blade) was used to cut a design into flesh. If the process was repeated or if a thorn was used to hook the flesh and pull it away from the body prior to the cut being made, then a more prominent, longer-lasting scar would have been achieved. Alternatively, if the open incision was rubbed with ash, earth, charcoal, indigo or the juice of berries, this irritant would also have produced a more vivid, raised scar.

Black skin is most likely to develop dramatic, prominent scar tissue (keloid) and it is interesting to speculate whether this is simply aesthetically fortuitous or if the early development of scarification in Africa – and in particular its equation with attractiveness and the resulting impact this may have had on sexual selection in this part of the world – actually contributed towards this physical trait becoming more pronounced among African peoples. Such speculation aside, what is clear is that the tendency of black skin to produce visually

MAKING DELIBERATE CUTS IN THE SKIN to produce designs of raised scar tissue, although far less popular than such other permanent body arts as tattooing and piercing, has found favour among an international minority of committed enthusiasts. *above left* Gzregorz, Poland, scarification made to enhance the line of the muscle; *above* Henk-Jan, Netherlands, horse scarification in the style of a cave painting; *opposite* Nicole, Netherlands, scarification on calves: the four ls, representing love, life, learning and lust

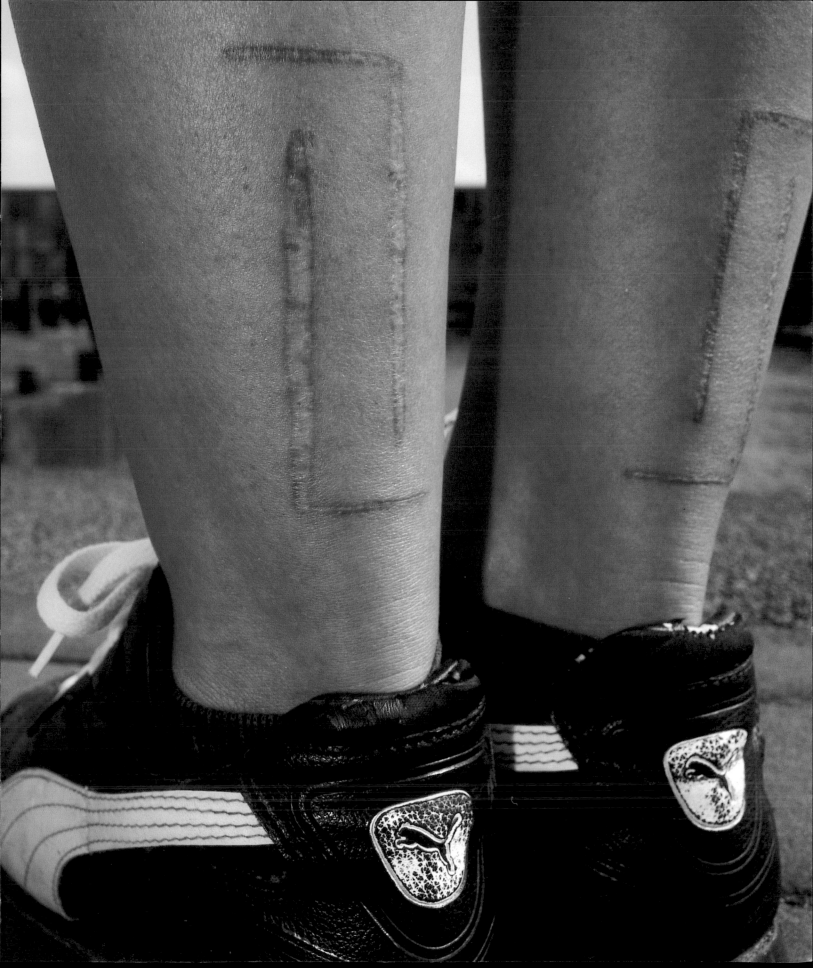

dramatic scar tissue made it a body art especially well-suited to the African continent, where a great variety of peoples employed it as a symbol of courage or endurance, a permanent mark of social identity, an irreversible indicator of passage through the different stages of life and, perhaps most significantly, the means by which a line could be drawn between the barbaric and the civilized. For, as the anthropologist Allen F. Roberts points out in *Marks of Civilization*, the word used by the Tabwa people of Zaire and Zambia for scarification – *kulemba* – is also their word for writing and bringing order and meaning to the world. Or, as the Baule people of the Ivory Coast see it, being scarred is an essential feature of being civilized.

I have written about scarification in Africa in the past tense because it is now disappearing from the continent where it was originally devised. Christian missionaries in Africa spoke out against it. Many African governments have banned such 'tribal marks'. And, increasingly, young people moving from the countryside to the cities have rejected this ancient practice as retrograde and unsophisticated.

Yet, although in decline among African peoples, there has in recent years been a significant increase of interest in scarification in Western culture. It would be inaccurate to suggest that it has penetrated the mainstream in the way that tattooing and piercing have, but, especially among Modern Primitives, there is a great attraction to this form of body decoration. Partly this is simply a result of tattooing and piercing becoming so popular and commonplace – prompting a need to look further afield for the unusual and distinctive.

More than this, however, scarification ('cutting' or cicatrization, as it is sometimes known) appeals to some people today precisely because of those characteristics that have in the past caused the majority to shun it: bloodletting and pain. For, as tribal peoples in Africa and elsewhere long appreciated, this form of body decoration carries a particularly powerful message of bravery, stoicism and perseverance. A man of the traditionally heavily scarred Tiv tribe in Nigeria told the anthropologist Paul Bohannan (also in *Marks of Civilization*): 'Of course it is painful. What girl would look at a man if his scars had not cost him pain?' As Bohannan goes on to explain, to the Tiv 'scarification, one of the finest decorations, is paid for in pain. The pain is proof positive that decoration is an unselfish act, and that it is done to give pleasure to others as well as oneself.' Contemporary interest in scarification has often

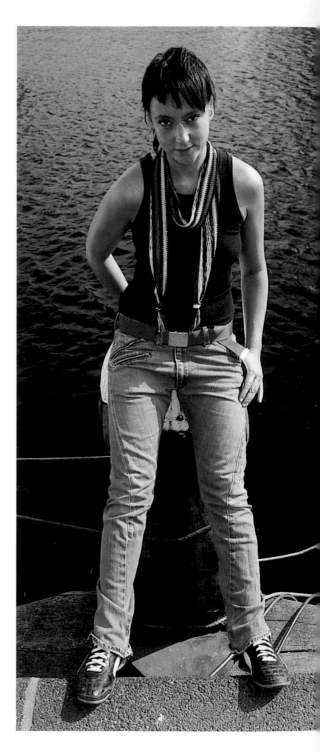

gone even beyond scars as a symbol of bravery – finding in the ritualistic experience of pain a transcendence of everyday reality; a purposeful exploration of self and being. It is, in other words, the process of acquiring such decorations – the ritual rather than the result – that is particularly valued by those who participate in what the American explorer/philosopher of Modern Primitive experience Fakir Musafar has termed 'body play'.

Many of those who have in recent years rediscovered scarification as body decoration and meaningful ritual have also explored the related phenomenon of branding (using heated metal to burn the skin). Once the mark of slaves and criminals in many cultures (including European), branding has particularly negative associations. It is also, obviously, extremely painful and a decorative technique of very limited subtlety. Yet, arguably even more so

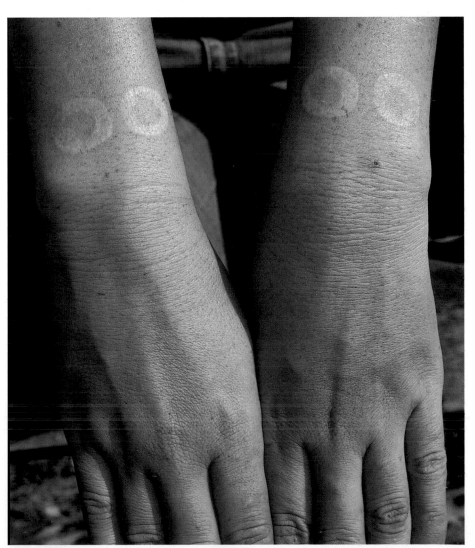

BRANDING IS A FAVOURED BODY DECORATION among a very small minority. Once used to mark slaves or criminals, part of its appeal today, as with scarification, is the painful, challenging ritual of its acquisition. *opposite* Nicole and *right* branding on her wrists

A CORE GROUP OF EXPERIMENTERS
has focused on less popular techniques of body decoration, now that tattooing and piercing are more commonplace, even mainstream and fashionable. *right* Dave at Tusk Tattoo & Body Piercing, with the game of noughts and crosses branded on his forearm and *below* scarification on his abdomen; *below right* Camilla, Brazil, with stainless steel implants in her arm

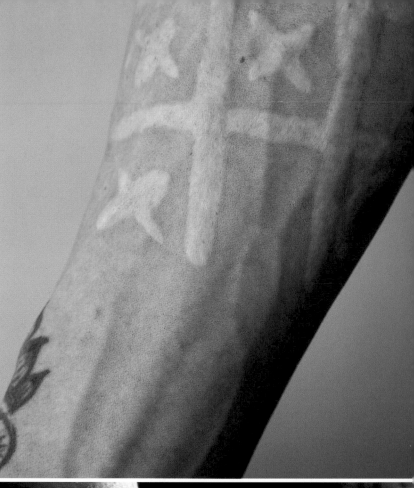

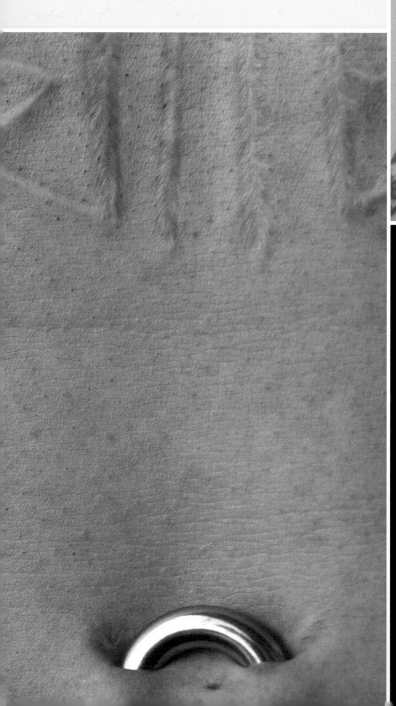

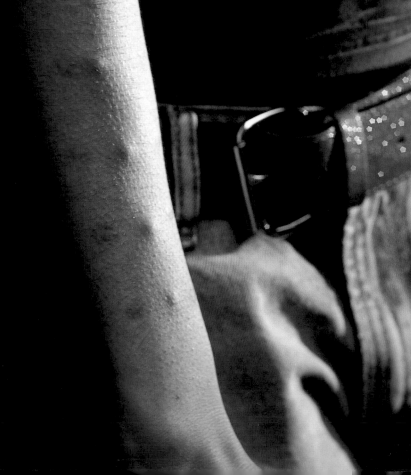

than scarification, its symbolic power is undeniable – as is evident in the erotic novel *The Story of O* when the heroine has her master's initials branded on her buttocks and, in a very different sense, in American universities, where the members of some predominantly black fraternities have branded themselves to demonstrate both their fortitude and lifelong commitment to their fraternity.

Another recent development in body decoration with clear links to scarification is the use of implants: the insertion of stainless steel, Teflon, coral, titanium, niobium, silicone and other objects under the skin to produce raised, tactile designs. This too has extensive and widespread historical antecedents. Many African cultures would place a small stone or similar object within a fresh scar so that, when healed over, the raised effect would be more dramatic and long-lasting. The ancient Maya of Central America often inserted pieces of bone, rings or coloured stones into a cut made in a man's penis – a practice paralleled more recently by some members of the Japanese Yakuza, who reportedly insert a pearl into the penis for each year served in prison.

Although long practised in Africa, the technique of implanting objects under the skin for three-dimensional decorative purposes is still a highly experimental form of body decoration in contemporary Western society. Obviously this is not something for the amateur to attempt him- or herself and few body piercers will openly admit that they carry out such work until they know the client personally and are convinced that they fully appreciate the extent to which this is a new technique that is not yet necessarily fully tested or indeed legal in some countries. Looking into the future, however, it is easy to imagine extraordinary developments in a body art that has the potential to transform the shape as well as the look of the body radically.

Taken together, scarification, branding and implants appear to offer a particularly extreme and striking new direction for body art today and in the future. The product of painful ritual (often valued as much as the resulting body decorations themselves), these techniques offer a creative option for a committed, dedicated minority who want to distance themselves from an increasingly tattooed and pierced mainstream.

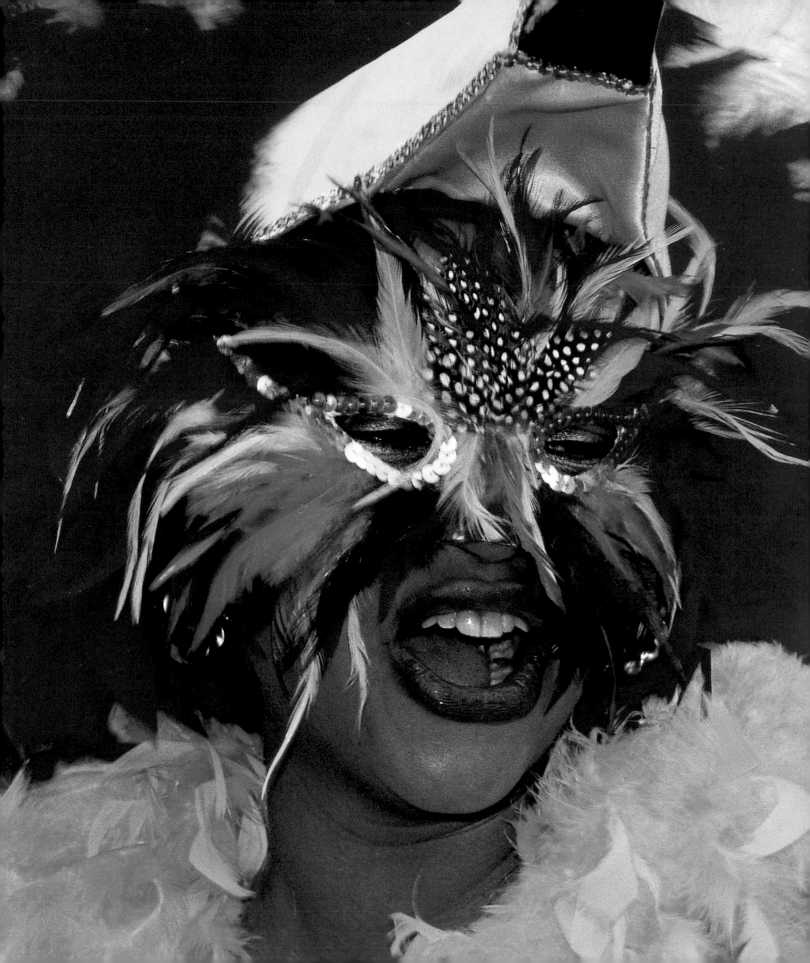

CHAPTER FOUR

THE ORNAMENTED BODY

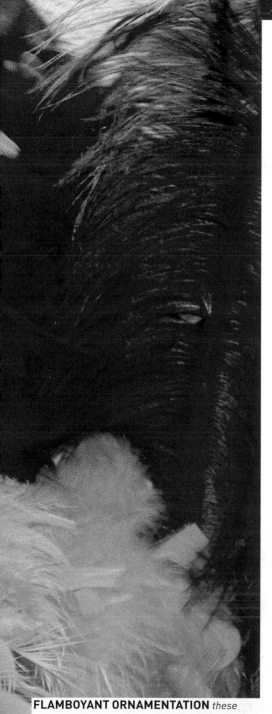

FLAMBOYANT ORNAMENTATION *these pages* mask and feathers, Carnival of Caribbean and South American Cultures, Rotterdam

An ornament is any object worn on, near or attached to the body. Usually we refer to such objects as jewelry, but this term doesn't conjure up images of flowers, leaves, twigs or feathers, which in all probability occupied a key place among the first ornaments – and which, from the Hawaiian tourist's floral necklace, the *Lei*, to a wedding corsage, remain important today. Although such fragile, impermanent materials have long since vanished from the archaeological record, their widespread use in traditional societies throughout the world points to their great antiquity.

Additionally, while the word 'jewelry' leads us to think in terms of particular, long-established classes of objects (earrings, necklaces, bracelets, rings and so forth) the term 'ornaments' opens a wider range of possibilities at a time when a new generation of designers is experimenting with interesting objects that fall outside of and defy the traditional, established ideas of jewelry. The term 'ornament' also helps us to appreciate the way in which objects that we carry on or near our bodies – glasses, sunglasses, mobile phones, pens, lighters, etc. – have, in addition to their 'real' functions, come to be coveted and scrutinized as ornaments. (Indeed, almost anything can be profitably considered an ornament – pets being a prime example – and in this sense it is interesting to hear of a craze in Japan for wearing fake bloodstained bandages.)

As well as all manner of found objects (shells, stones, animal teeth, gourds, parts of insects, bones as well as the

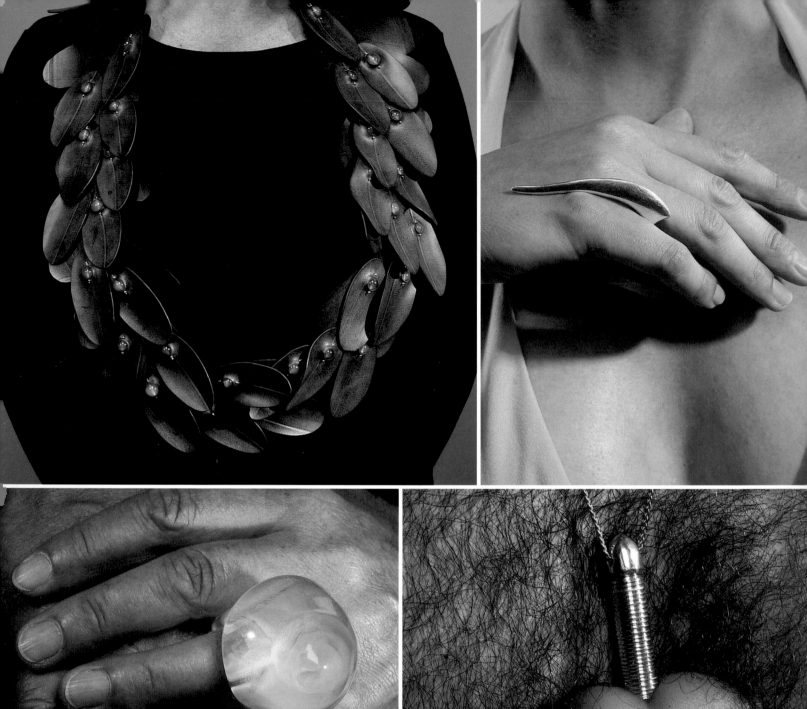

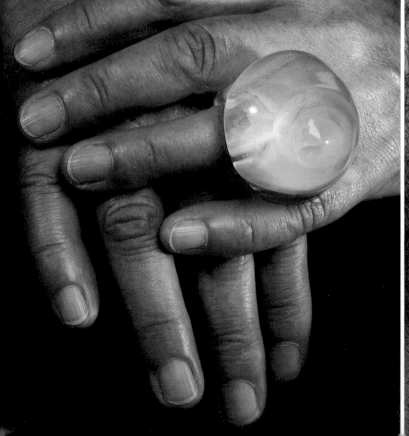

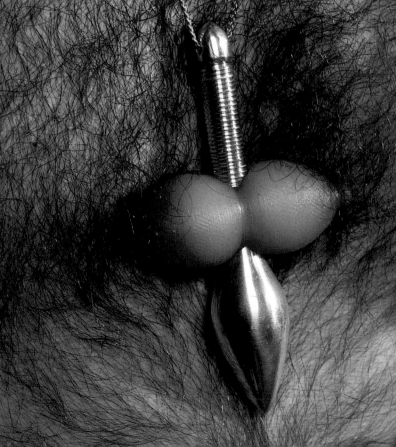

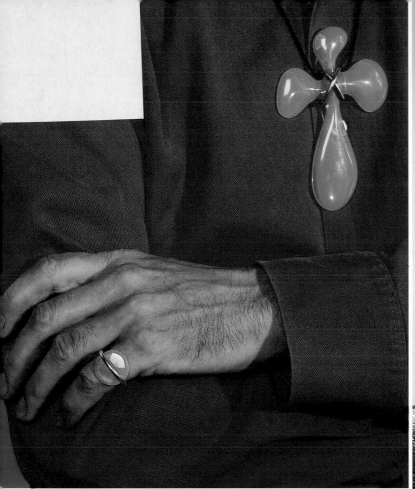

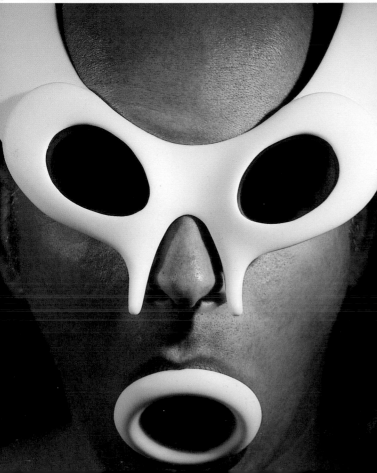

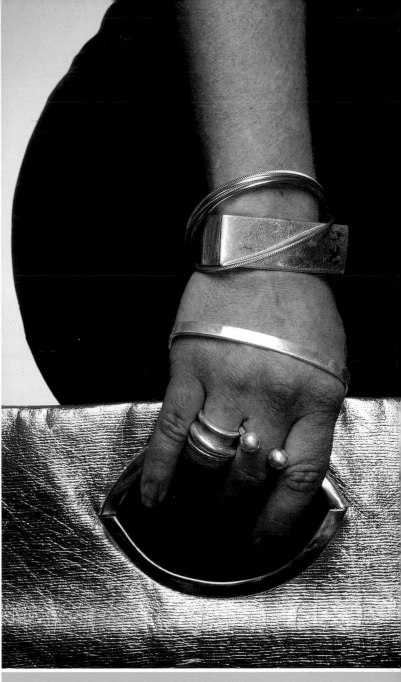

AN EXCITING TIME FOR JEWELRY DESIGN,
new materials are being introduced and the relationship
between ornament and the body is re-explored. *from
top left, clockwise*: Miecke, wearing laurel-leaf necklace
made from car parts (rubber inner tubes) and precious
stones, by Thea Tolsma; Lianne wearing finger piece
by Naomi Filmer; Paul Derrez wearing a crucifix and
ring of his own design, in aluminium and nylon; Josie
wearing modern silver jewelry including hand piece by
Johanna Reiss; Jaap wearing mask and mouth tube
by Florian Ladstätter; Paul Derrez wearing 'Australian
Tits' pendant of his own design; Miecke wearing epoxy
ring by Wim van Doorschodt

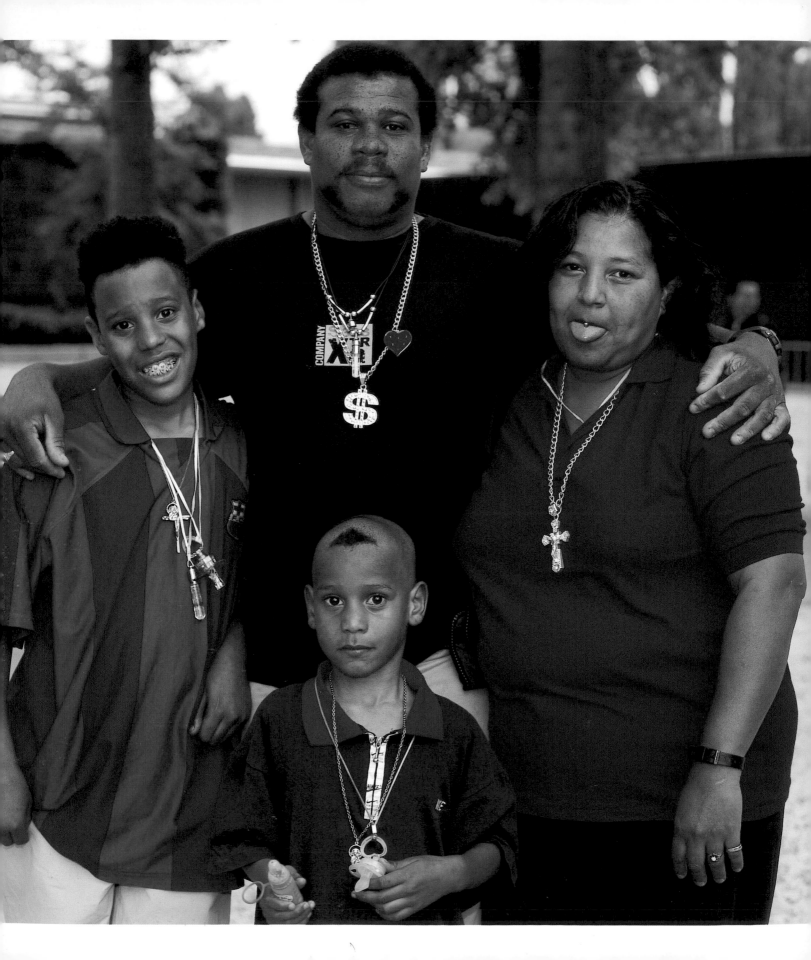

ORNAMENTS ARE COMMUNICATION DEVICES,
as well as having aesthetic value. *opposite left to right*
Randy Junior, Randy, Dorian and Rujuwen (*front*),
a truly decorated family, celebrating God and money;
below Arabic script name necklace

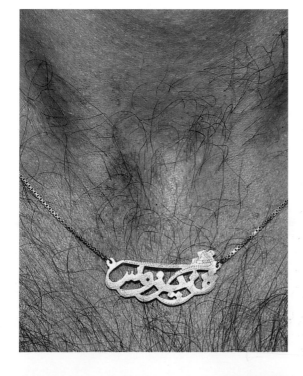

aforementioned flowers, leaves, twigs and feathers) human beings have made use of every available technology to manufacture ornaments to display on their bodies. A history of such adornment is also a history of humankind's technological development: from the shaping of stones, the carving of tusk, bone or wood and various discoveries in metalworking through to more recent advances in plastics and other synthetic materials. It is difficult to think of any object or material that hasn't been used somewhere, at some time, for adorning the body. Indeed, this hunger for new styles of ornament may have played a significant role in pushing forward technological progress throughout history.

Dictionary definitions of ornaments inevitably describe such objects as 'decorative' and with only a few, minor exceptions (for example, objects worn in battle to frighten the enemy, or deliberately disturbing masks) this is usually the case: people create and wear such objects because they see them as beautiful; something that will make them look more attractive. But to view such objects as merely decorative is to fail to appreciate the significant, sometimes vital functions that the vast majority of ornaments serve beyond simply looking nice.

Whether the amulets worn by the Taureg of Niger (which contain verses from the Quran or ancient magical formulas), a rabbit's foot or a St Christopher medal, many ornaments have been worn because of the protective powers they are seen to possess. In all probability such talismans have been a key part of the history of ornament from the very beginning. In general, people today dismiss the idea of ornaments as magical, but from the charm bracelet to the Queen's crown (the symbol of her power) and the Christian cross (even if ostensibly worn as a marker of religious affiliation, rather than as a talisman per se, still capable of incinerating vampires on sight in horror movies) it is clear that we still, even if subconsciously, credit some ornaments with powers beyond that of logical expectation.

In many parts of the world ornaments are not only valuable, they are (or were) the only known currency and means of preserving wealth from one generation to the next and an insurance against hard times. As such wealth is often the property of women, it can create an important counterbalance to the economic power of men. Such wearable wealth, however, also has its disadvantages, as can be seen, for example, in parts of Africa, where the size and weight of metal anklets or bracelets may constitute a terrible and lifelong burden.

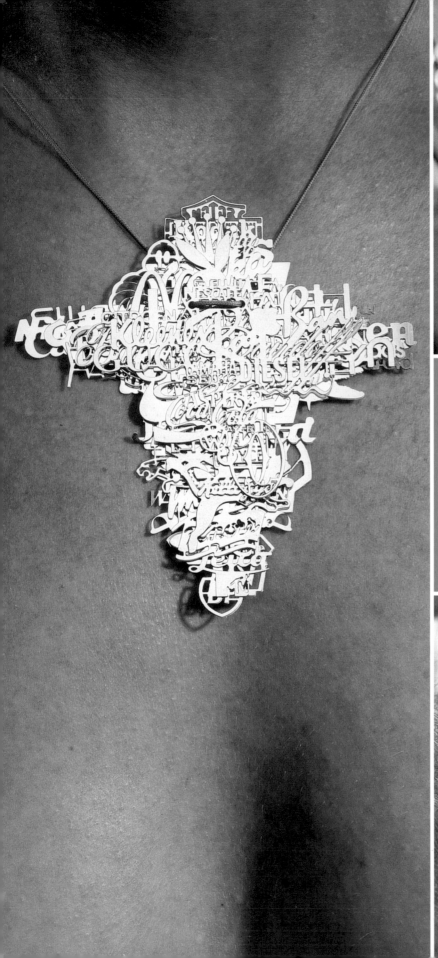

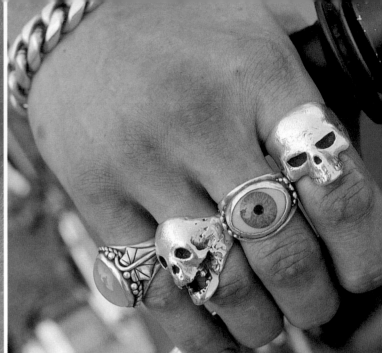

STATUS, WEALTH, ROLE, RELIGIOUS BELIEFS,
lifestyle and philosophy – like all forms of body
decoration, ornament often serves to communicate
information about those who wear it. Even when
widely understood, symbolism is often deliberately
subverted. *left* Lianne wears 'bling bling' crucifix by
Frank Tjepkema, a design using religious iconography
to comment on streetstyle reverence towards wealth
and brand names; *above* Jake, wearing Great Frog
silver Rocker-boy rings; *below* Gzregorz wears a
fake Rolex watch

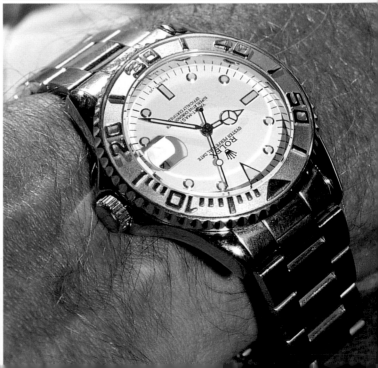

Some ornaments (like most clothing) provide modest concealment that is capable of transforming the naked into the respectable. While a differing cultural definition of modesty may make it difficult for Westerners to appreciate, for many traditional peoples it remains the case that to be seen in public without earrings, beaded belt or anklets brings the same shame or embarrassment a Westerner would feel if caught without clothing in public. In a similar way, the penis sheaths made from large gourds (and anything from bamboo, ivory, wood, shells and animal horn to metal) that were worn by tribal men in many parts of the Amazon, the south-west Pacific and Africa, while on first sight provocative, boastful masculine display, actually served the purpose of modest concealment and the social control of sexual inclination as Peter Ucko (in the definitive work on the subject, 'Penis Sheaths: A Comparative Study') concludes: 'penis sheaths in most societies have remarkably few phallic connotations and are rather, symbols of modesty and decorum...The sheath is [in most societies] not simply a symbol of sexual maturity but one of social control of that sexuality. The penis sheath, in many instances, is not primarily a sexual symbol in itself but a visible sign of sexual restriction.'

As this quote makes clear, while the penis sheath may literally conceal male genitals and actually restrict sexual behaviour, its real power is symbolic. And this is indeed the primary, most universal, most fundamental and most indispensable function of all forms of adornment: visual communication. As the anthropologist Ian Tattersall suggests in *The Monkey in the Mirror*, this has always been the case: the bracelets, pendants, necklaces and other ornaments found among Cro-Magnon burial remains (some thirty to forty thousand years old) are an important indication of the symbol-centred revolution that defined the first Homo sapiens as unique and separate from all other creatures. To decorate the body with found or specially crafted objects is to transform it into a meaningful system – a language.

But what does ornament say? From the North American Indian chief's elaborate headdress to Western wedding or engagement rings, ornaments serve to signal social role and status. Likewise, Western use of ornament as a display of wealth (the pearl necklace, the huge diamond ring, the Rolex watch, designer sunglasses, etc.) has been present throughout human history (or at least since the development of economic hierarchies).

In today's world the language of ornament is at least as important as it has ever been, but increasingly what we intend it to 'say' about us is quite different from what our ancestors 'said'. There is an increasing trend towards ornaments designed to signal that the wearer is a unique, multifaceted individual who stands out from the amorphous mass – interesting objects signalling an interesting person. In this context the meanings of ornaments become more complex and subtle; more difficult to pinpoint and define. But far from diminishing the importance of ornament today, its ever-increasing communicative subtlety and sophistication – ornaments serving as adjectives of attitude, values, lifestyle and personal direction – seems certain to make it an ever more valuable, indispensable form of self-expression.

The human body naturally provides lots of different, useful places for the attachment of objects – the neck, wrists, ankles and waist offer particular security. But human beings have also put headdresses on their heads, rings on their fingers, strapped ornaments over their feet or hands and around their elbows, biceps, thighs or knees, tightened headbands around foreheads, fitted masks over faces, positioned glasses using the bridge of the nose and the ears, pinned brooches to their clothing, glued false eyelashes over eyelids, clamped hats on heads, fastened fabric patches or gemstones onto skin, wedged flowers behind their ears, stuck all manner of things in their hair and held sceptres and ornamental fans (or today, specially styled mobile phones) in their hands.

Yet, perpetually dissatisfied by even this wide range of possibilities, human beings have devised other, more permanent means of attaching objects to their bodies. For example, many peoples found ways of embedding precious stones or metals in their teeth (a practice brought to a considerable standard of achievement in ancient Mesoamerican civilizations that still flourishes today in many parts of the world – most famously among hip hop musicians). But the most universal and widespread technique of permanently attaching decorative objects to the body – found on every continent and throughout history – is that of piercing holes through flesh.

Thorns, sticks, bamboo spikes and sharp splinters of bone were the precursors of the piercing guns and hollow needles that are used today. Historically, the sites on the body most favoured for piercing were the septum and nostrils of the nose, areas around the lips (for example the labret adornments of many Inuit groups), the rim of the ear and the earlobe (so apparently purpose-built for this

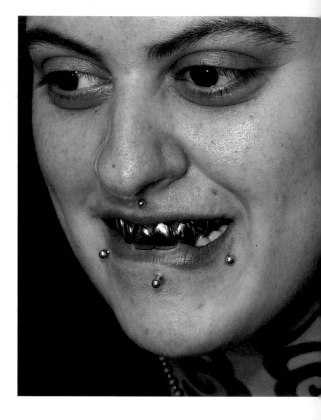

DECORATING THE TEETH,
as well as skin and hair, has a long human history. This has taken the form of filing them into points, staining their colour or – from the Aztecs to today's hip hop stars – embedding or replacing them with precious metals or stones. *above* Roxx at Eyegasm Tattoo, with metal teeth, multiple piercings and tattoos: 'Beauty in the eye of this beholder is transforming perfect, straight teeth into bling bling chrome plates. Now I love my teeth!'; *opposite* Jake shows off his gold teeth

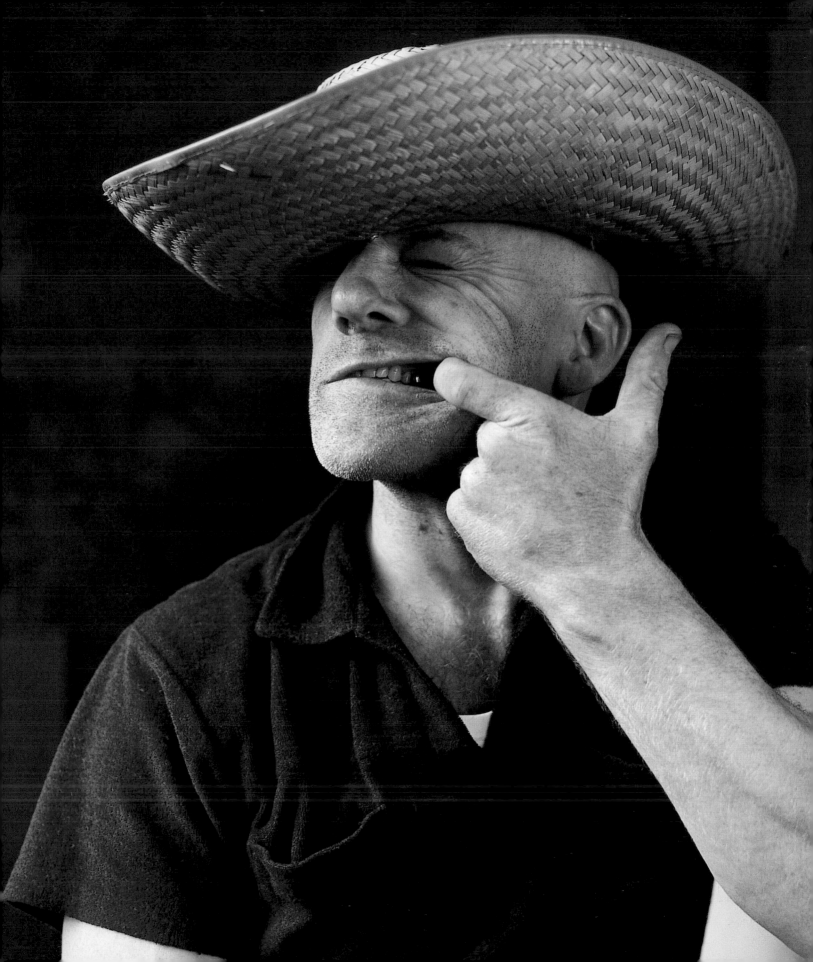

role that one can't help but wonder if this otherwise seemingly useless bit of flesh didn't evolve specifically for decorative reasons). Some traditional peoples also devised piercings for the genitals – the *ampallang* side to side through the head of the penis in Borneo; the *apadravya* that passes through the head of the penis from front to back in southern India; and the *guiche* piercing of the rim of flesh behind the scrotum in many parts of the South Pacific. Although the recent piercing renaissance has often (and rightly) been seen as a revival of primitive techniques, many of the most popular piercings of today (for example, the navel, the tongue, the nipples, all piercings for the female genitals) are unusual or completely unknown in traditional societies.

However, stretched piercings – where the size of the pierced hole is gradually increased, often to astonishing proportions – have a legitimate primitive pedigree. Indeed, even among the most extreme of today's Modern Primitives few if any have yet matched the accomplishments of such peoples as the Surma of south-western Ethiopia or the Suya of the Amazon. While it is the men of the Suya tribe who stretch initially small piercings in their lips to accommodate wooden discs the size of CDs, it is the women of the Surma who practise this technique of body modification: prior to marriage a lip piercing is fitted with ever larger wooden or clay plates – the 'bride price' paid by the groom's family to the bride's family is then calculated on the size of her eventual (round or wedge-shaped) plug.

The stretching of earlobes to amazing size was found in a great many traditional societies including, most famously, the elite of Easter Island in the Pacific, whose long, pendant-like lobes are clearly seen on the huge stone statues that this culture left to posterity. While few if any people today have lip piercings stretched to the extent practised by the likes of the Suya and the Surma, stretched earlobes – often with an internal ring inserted to maintain the shape of the hole, another technique deriving from traditional societies – are common. Probably unique to Western culture, there are some who have used piercing to stretch the length of their nipples and labia.

Few things are so astounding today as regards appearance and style in the West as the speed and the extent to which piercing has been transformed from an adornment technique used only for the earlobes and only by women (and the odd sailor) into a mainstream phenomenon for both women and men (and, it should be pointed out, a particularly exciting genre of jewelry design). As

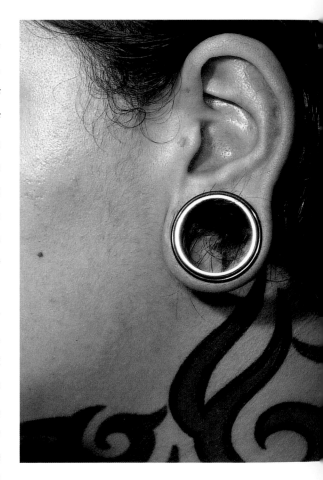

AN INITIAL PIERCING MAY BE STRETCHED to enormous size, as tribal peoples discovered long ago. Today's Modern Primitives have revived this body art for the ear lobe but, at least so far, shown little interest in the huge, CD-sized lip plates found in parts of the Amazon and Africa. *above* Roxx at Eyegasm Tattoo, inspired by 'ethnic tribal peoples and global culture', with stretched ear piercing by Sean Henderson (neck tattoos by William del Ray and Marty Maaske)

with the tattoo renaissance, this revival has its historical roots principally in the West Coast of America. In particular, Doug Malloy found himself attracted – even obsessed, by his own account – to these ancient body-art techniques, and used his training in anthropology to explore its development in Borneo, New Guinea and Tahiti. Freely experimenting on his own body, Malloy gained a basic knowledge of many of these techniques, which he then passed on to friends such as Jim Ward (founder of Gauntlet and *Piercing Fans International Quarterly* [*PFIQ*] magazine) and Mr Sebastian (one of Britain's great piercing pioneers).

Malloy, Ward and Mr Sebastian were all gay men and, at least initially, the primary impact of their work was in the gay community. Also experimenting with piercing and other forms of body play in California, Fakir Musafar invented the concept of Modern Primitives, which (especially when it became the title of an extremely popular book that features interviews with Musafar and others) brought interest in piercing to a demographically broader group. But the Western piercing renaissance also owes a great debt to the non-professionals of Punk who (with not-to-be-recommended disregard for hygiene and infection) thrust safety pins and other sharp objects through their faces as an expression of a 'tribal' mindset and as a definitively shocking gesture.

It is a big jump from the influential but minority confines of some circles within the gay community, sartorially extreme Punks and the originally tiny world of the first Modern Primitives to the mainstream phenomenon we see today, in which young people from Japan to the USA, Britain to Russia now see an eyebrow, septum, tongue, lip, labret or navel piercing as normal, even *de rigueur*. Part of the explanation for this has already been introduced within our discussion on tattooing: the shift away from change for its own sake to the continuity offered by permanent body decoration; the attractions of what is seen as 'street' and authentic over the merely fashionable.

We should also consider here the element of meaningful ritual that the short, sharp shock of piercing particularly epitomizes. That is to say, the appeal of piercing today may not only be the decorative possibilities it provides but – perhaps even more so – the painful process it requires. For countless traditional peoples piercing offered a particularly focused ritual moment; a rite of passage that, in one sharp moment of pain, transforms a child into an adult. Something similar occurs even today in scattered rural parts of Europe: an Irish friend has

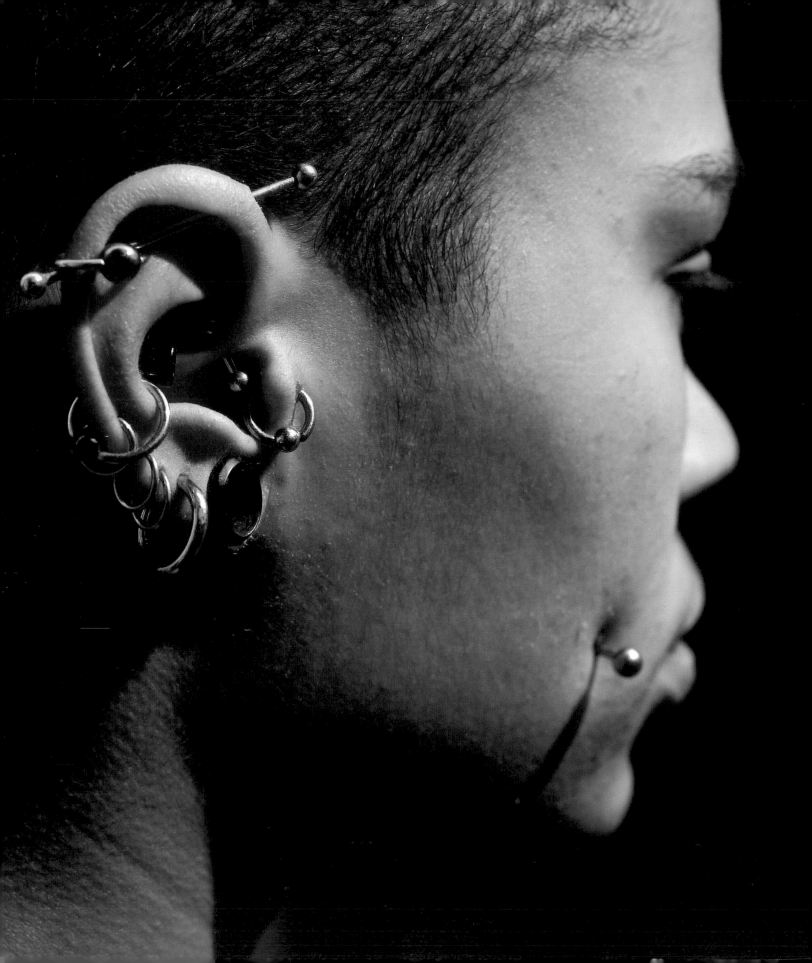

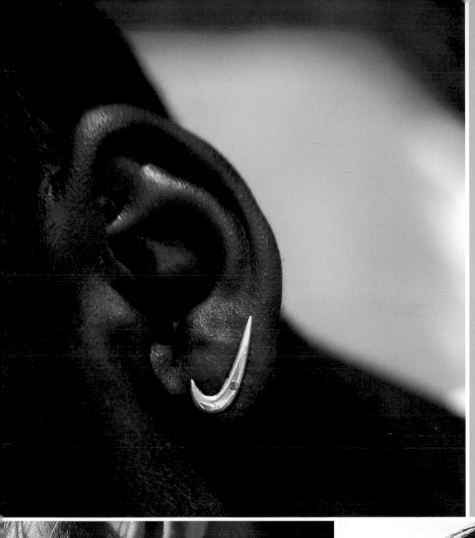

PIERCING TODAY IS POSTMODERN

in flavour. One of the most ancient forms of body decoration, with the exception of pierced ear lobes (and usually only for women) it was long seen as 'barbaric' and bizarre in the West. Now, not only are facial and body piercings acceptable, at least in certain circles, they are *de rigueur*. *opposite* Camilla, Brazil, multiple ear piercings and cheek stud; *left* Cuban piercing jewelry imitates the Nike swoosh; *below* Rui, Portugal, juxtaposition of traditional piercings with distinctly contemporary ornaments – a combination of sunglasses, neckpiece and piercings; *below left* Kor Klompsma, Netherlands, wearing jewelry of his own design

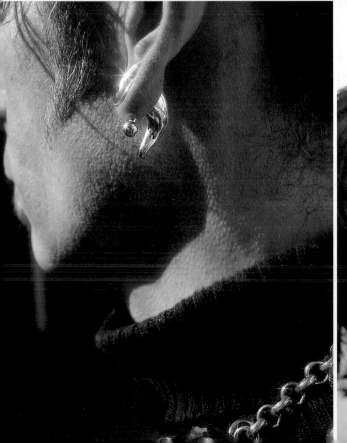

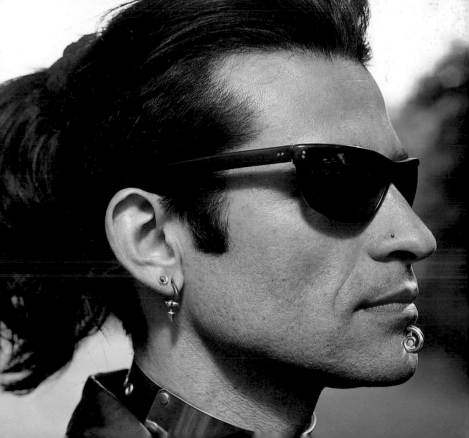

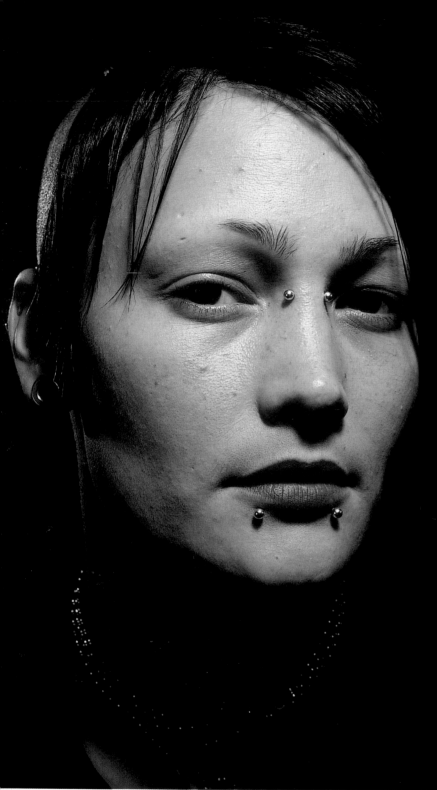

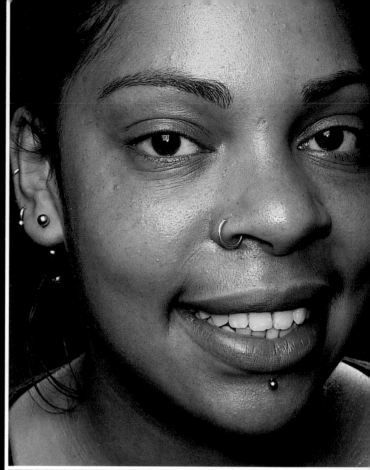

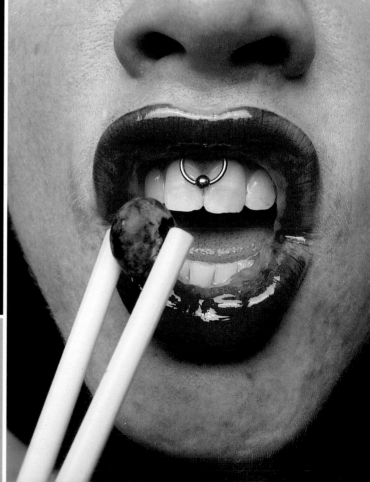

EVEN FIFTY YEARS AGO,
no one would have believed the extent to which
all manner of piercings have become a common,
even ubiquitous sight in contemporary culture.
above Anja, lip, bridge and ear piercings;
above right Gracia, nose ring, lip stud and multiple
ear piercings; *right* Josie, frenum piercing

described to me how in the small farming community where she grew up, a girl would be taken to have her ears pierced as soon as she began menstruating.

Contemporary urban and suburban culture, however, as part of a general shift away from all forms of ritual, has banished as barbarous the ancient notion of a physical rite of passage. Without these rituals people's lives are often empty, lacking in meaning and demarcation, and nowhere is this more evident than in Western teens, who seem dazed and confused by the ambiguity of their social status. Neither children nor adults, hungry for a significant ritual to mark officially their transformation to adulthood, one reason for the extraordinary popularity of piercing might be that it provides (even if self-imposed) a powerful, focused occasion when ordinary life recedes to the fringes of consciousness (which is what ritual aims to accomplish) to herald a transformation, a rite of passage.

The ritual of piercing can serve to mark all manner of moments of personal transformation (its use at the start or the end of a relationship also seems to be increasingly popular). It is also true that, although the action of getting a piercing is particularly focusing for the obvious reason of the pain, the moment of acquiring any ornament even without piercing can be ritually powerful and transformative. The exchange of rings at a wedding ceremony and the coronation of a monarch are good examples of how acquiring an ornament can serve to signal a fundamental change in personal status – putting the ornament on is a significant ritual moment, a passage from one state into another.

One class of ornament – the mask – is not only explicitly transformative, but can also serve symbolically to identify and express what those who put them on have (even if only temporarily) become. Today – the likes of Batman, Zorro, swag-laden thieves and stocking-covered gunmen predominating in Western mental associations – people tend to think of masks only as a mechanism of concealment; simply a way of obliterating personal identity to achieve anonymity. Although there is some historic and ethnographic precedent for this usage (for example the masks worn by the members of the 'secret societies' of some African and Pacific cultures, which allow judgment to be passed on wrongdoers without the judges incurring personal responsibility), the primary function of masks throughout history and in most societies has been more positive – revealing in the action of concealing. As such, masks are one of humankind's most magical, extraordinary inventions – transformation machines that mirror the quality of human consciousness that permits not only the realization 'I am' but also the realization that I could be other than what I am. (Or, indeed, the awareness that I am many different things simultaneously. For, as Anthony Shelton points out in his discussion of Mexican masks in John Mack's *Masks and the Art of Expression*, other cultures have had more fluid and inclusive – arguably more liberating and healthy – notions of the boundaries between being human, animal and spirit.)

A mask makes it possible for one person to become another person, an animal, a spirit, a god, a mythic or theatrical character, a different gender, the embodiment of a particular emotion and, in temporarily casting aside the particularity of personal identity, to become a generalized role model. While all these usages are ancient, they also have applications in the world today – whether at a Hallowe'en party, a carnival procession or a fetish club.

In the West people tend to see such masquerading as 'just a bit of fun', but the escape from self and the role-playing that masks allow us is, as our ancestors well knew, a valuable (arguably essential) ritual means of exploring and understanding ourselves, our fears, dreams and desires. Contemporary psychology often seems to suggest that in order to truly know ourselves we must peel away the masks we hide behind; but as it conceals, the mask has magical powers to reveal – powers that might be useful within the context of the contemporary Postmodern crises of identity and meaning.

As with tattooing, the West has often seen masks and masquerading as something that was taken seriously only by other, exotic (Africa, Oceania, Japan) or very ancient cultures (Egypt, Greece and Rome). In truth, masks played a significant, often crucial part in ritual life in Europe up to (and in a surprising range of places, including) the present day. As Cesare Poppi points out in 'The Other Within: Masks and Masquerades in Europe', both in pagan and Christian eras a powerful correspondence existed between the seasonal transitions of winter and summer and the use of masks in ordering and controlling the problematic relationship between the living and the dead. In particular, it is interesting that Hallowe'en was originally the date of the Celtic New Year: the point being that in such transitional moments, when the earth itself is reborn, life is precarious and inherently dangerous and masks make it possible to confront these fears and triumph over them. Christianity often sought to suppress traditions of masquerading, but failed as its own celebration of rebirth (Easter)

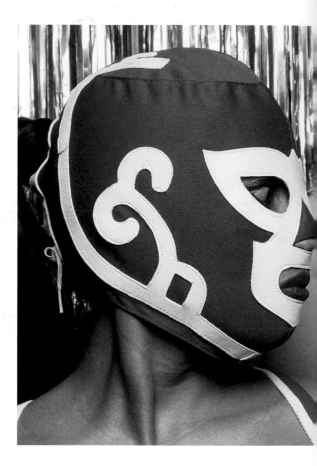

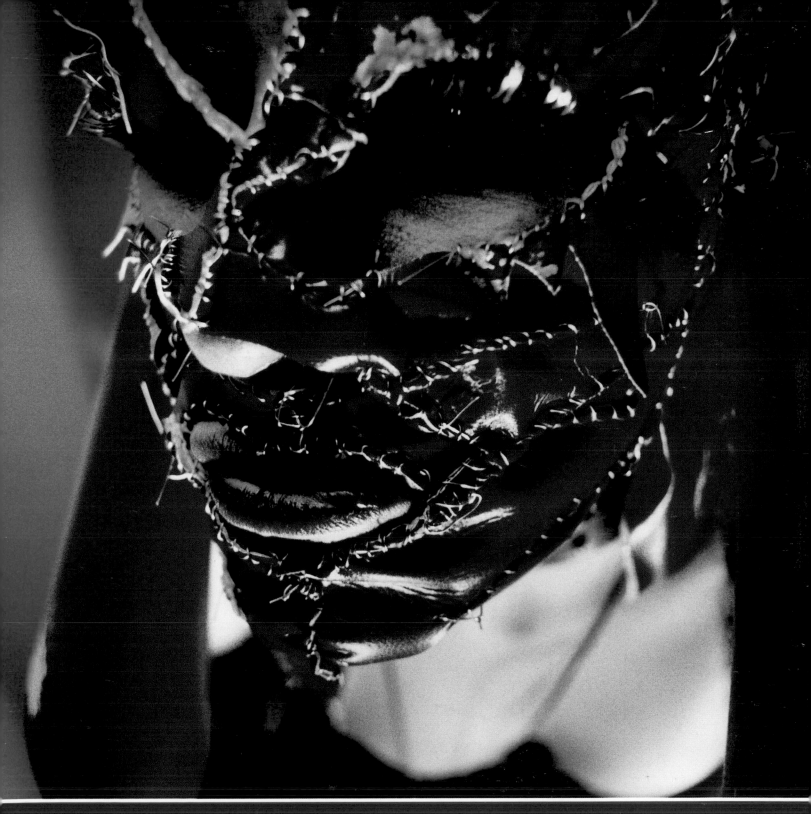

FAR FROM JUST A BIT OF FUN,
masks offer a supreme opportunity for experimenting with changes of personal
identity. As our ancestors knew and as we are now rediscovering, these magical
transformation machines can reveal alternative, inner selves at the same time as they
provide anonymity. *opposite* Joan, wearing Mexican wrestling mask; *above* Maureen,
in handmade PVC and patent leather mask, which she has sewn and stapled together

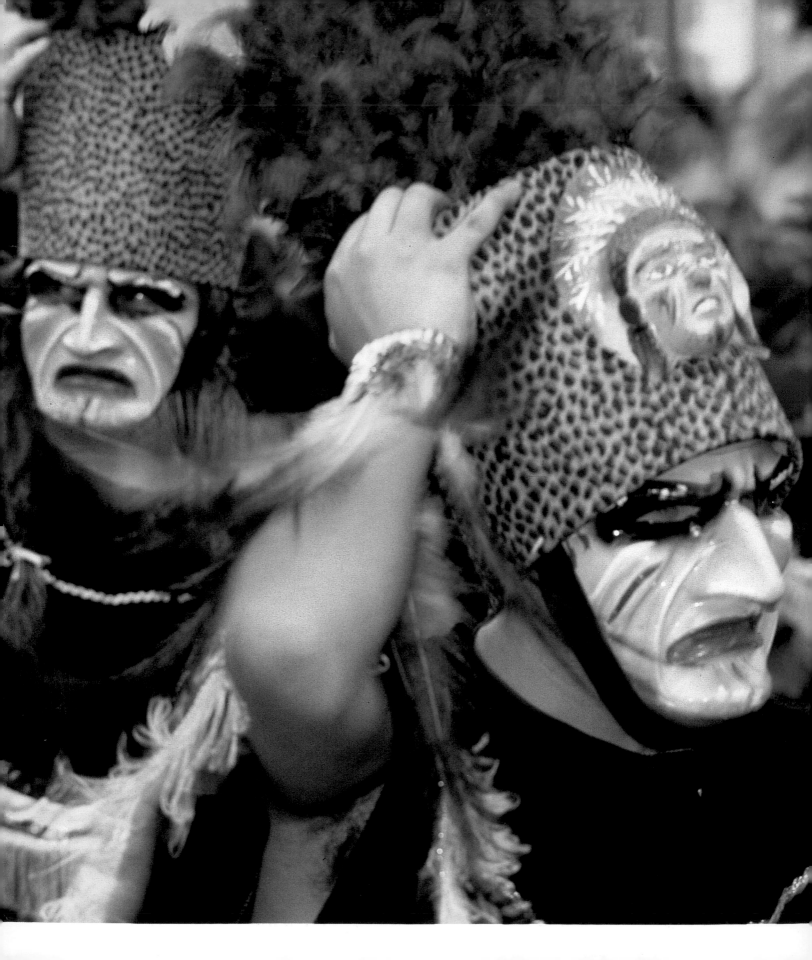

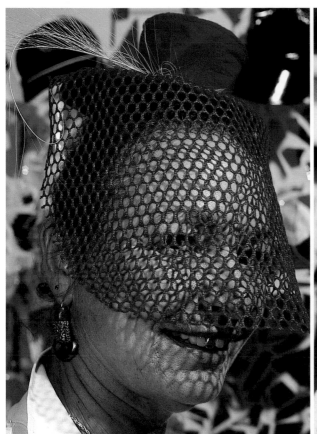

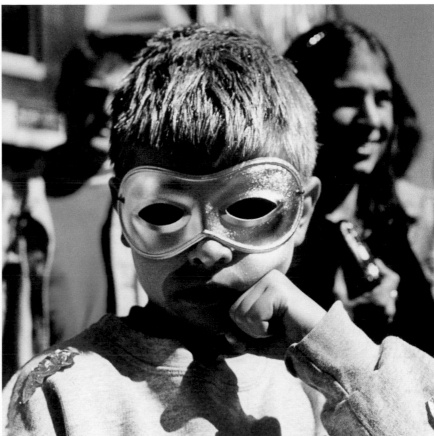

became the occasion of carnival – which, from Rio to Venice, New Orleans to Notting Hill in London, remains the other great masquerading event in Western culture. Indeed, even a masked figure such as Harlequin (who today is associated simply with comic playfulness and presumed to be only as old as the *Commedia dell'arte* of the 16th and 17th centuries), is actually the representation of one of Europe's oldest and most widespread mythic characters: the leader of the marching army of the dead, which appears at transitional times in the seasonal calendar.

The ancient – sinister but ultimately restorative – legacy of masks suggests that, like so many forms of ornament, they continue to be invaluable tools for exploring human nature and possibility. In the film *The Mask*, Jim Carrey's character eventually throws the magical metamorphosis machine back into the water, but let us not forget that this ornament has done its job: permitting a mere mortal to realize the god-like powers within himself. The transformative power of masks is particularly explicit but, in truth, all ornament – far from simply looking nice – has the possibility of changing as well as articulating who we are.

THE POWER TO TRANSFORM
the wearer is common to all ornaments, but particularly evident in the case of masks. This quality makes masks useful for underlining the magical nature of ritual events – from carnival to one's wedding day. *opposite* mask-wearing participants at the Carnival of Caribbean and South American Cultures, Rotterdam; *above* Ans at Pet Salon Milliners wears hat and veil she was married in; *above right* boy at street party in face paint and mask

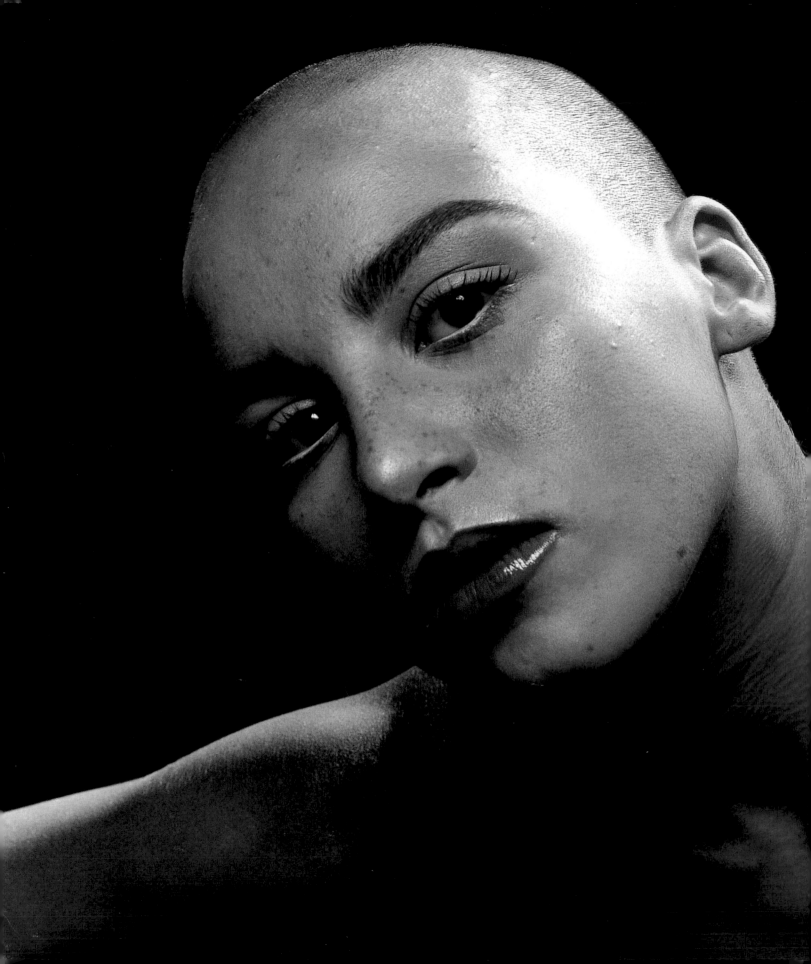

THE HAIRY BODY

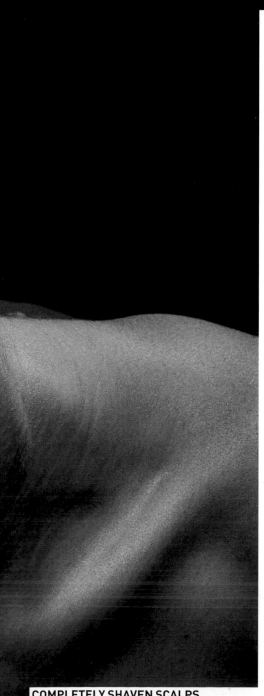

COMPLETELY SHAVEN SCALPS
on women are one of the most striking
hairstyles of recent years. *these pages* Nadia

Nails and hair occupy a unique – even strange – position on the edge of our physical selves. They are a part of us but at the same time they are continually in the process of departing from us, in a journey from the subjective to the objective; from the living to the dead. It is this very ambiguity that makes them fascinating, powerful and potentially disturbing. The stuff of both dreams and nightmares, they remind us that we have within ourselves beasts (werewolves, all hairy and clawed), which we fear may at any moment burst through our thin veneer of civilization and restraint. Contained within this fear is a hope that (at least in bed) we retain some vestige of our animal selves. Yet, when carefully groomed, nails and hair also become symbols of civilized sophistication. Like fur and feathers, nails and hair are made of the protein keratin and built-in obsolescence is central to their design. Always in the process of regeneration, they are at the same time always in the process of dying. Yet even when they have broken away or been deliberately cut off from our bodies, these disposable body parts – at least in our mind's eye – retain their intimate, personal associations.

Sometimes these associations are positive: for example the cherished lock of hair of a distant or departed loved one that the Victorians mounted in frames or wove into watch chains or necklaces. Alexander Pope's mock-epic poem 'The Rape of the Lock' recounts the true story of how two English families entered into a seemingly unending feud when Lord Petre succumbed to 'the irresistible lure of the lock' and

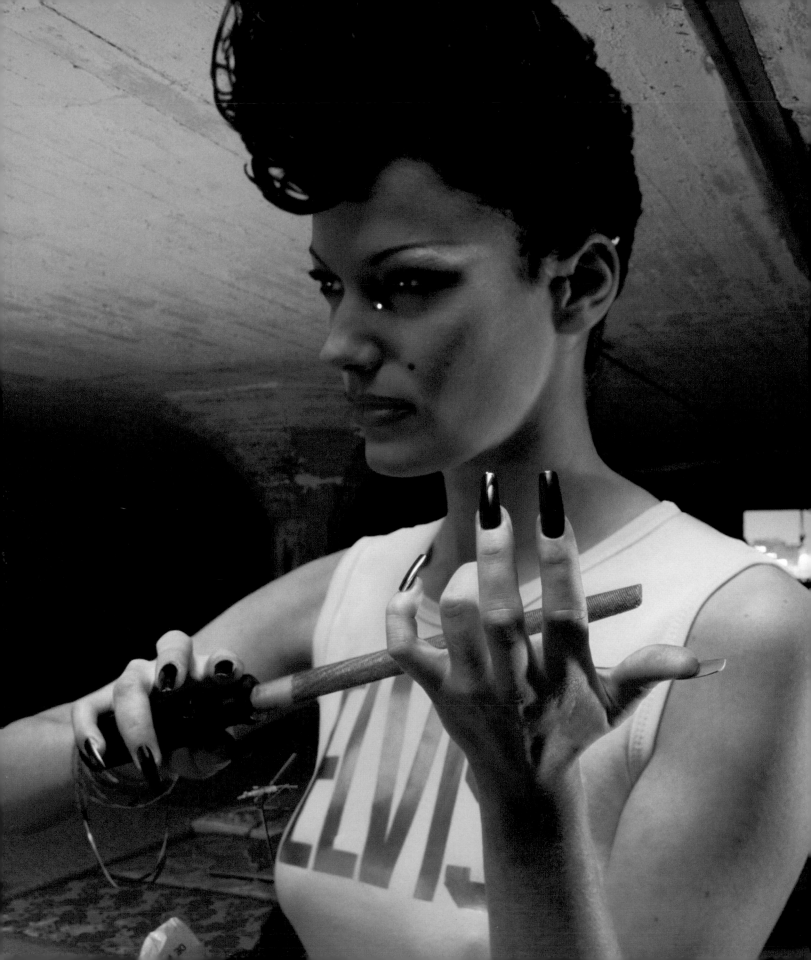

snipped off a bit of Miss Arabella Fermor's hair. When African slaves were sold and families wrenched apart by New World plantation owners it was often a single lock of hair that served as a symbolic link between parents and children, husbands and wives. Traditionally at Korean weddings the groom wore a hat woven from the hair clippings of his father's ancestors. In the Malagasy Republic, now Madagascar, it was once the custom that, after a child's first, ritual haircut, the clippings would be mixed with food and eaten by family and guests. The Tzotzil women of Mexico saved their hair clippings so that, after death, these would become a rope to take them to heaven. But throughout human history the intrinsic power possessed by hair and nail clippings has also made them objects to be feared. Given their intimate associations with the person they came from, such clippings could be used in sorcery. For this reason, many if not most traditional societies disposed of them carefully in secret by burial or burning. The same was true in the West, as it was thought that a witch could use such clippings to gain control over someone. Today we are more nonchalant about these matters but our (largely irrational) loathing of such materials – the horror of finding a stray hair or nail clipping in a hotel bathroom for example – suggests that we still retain a sense of their power.

While sharing this me/not me, alive/(un)dead status, nails and hair have had very different histories in terms of their decoration. Very simply, this is because of the daily hardship imposed on nails by manual labour. Except for the most rudimentary colouring (for example with henna) there is little in the way of nail decoration in tribal or peasant societies. It was only with the development of social hierarchies in which an upper class became exempt from manual labour that more sophisticated forms of nail art were able to develop. Within such elites, however, decoration of the nails has always had a particularly important role as a marker of status. Indeed, even without artful decoration, very long and/or perfectly manicured nails are incontestable proof that a person can afford to have others do their dirty work.

Aside from occasionally colouring the nails and, in some Asian cultures, extending them with delicately curved metal tips (as worn by some oriental dancers to accentuate hand movement), decoration of the nails only really took off as an art in recent times. In the 1930s, Charles and Joseph Revson's Revlon company shot to success with the introduction of the first commercially available nail enamels (using pigments rather than dyes to produce more vivid and

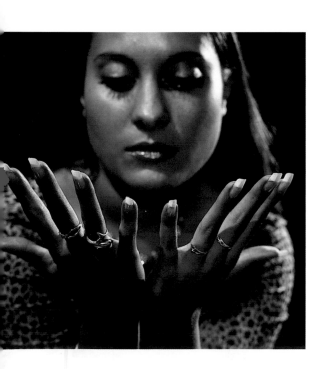

LONG, CAREFULLY MANICURED NAILS
have always been a status symbol – proof that one doesn't have to engage in strenuous manual labour. New techniques for creating huge, artificial extensions, an ever-widening range of colours, and creative innovations in design have made nail art one of the most exciting and rapidly advancing body decoration techniques. *opposite* Marie-Louise, with hair extensions pinned to her quiff and false nails; *above* Magda, with natural but distinctively manicured long nails

longer-lasting colours). By the end of the 1930s, Revlon had also begun to introduce new colours with each fashion season and matching shades for nails and lipstick. As dramatic as these changes were at the time – with not only Hollywood actresses but, more often than not, the average housewife suddenly sporting colourful fingers and toes – they were eclipsed towards the end of the 20th century by an extraordinary nail art revolution. This was triggered by technological advances that made enormous, long-lasting nail extensions possible and by the creativity and imagination of the artists who worked in the nail salons that mushroomed in America and Britain, especially in black communities. Whether an ever changing range of airbrushed mini-masterpiece designs or its experiments with futuristic, crystal-clear acrylic talons that explode with colour only at the tip, nail art is arguably today's most rapidly advancing form of body decoration. Creative and scientific advances aside, the nail art revolution of recent years could not have happened without the fact that social, economic and technological factors have meant that huge numbers of people in developed societies today can avoid the sort of manual labour that previously made this body decoration impossible but for a tiny elite.

Hair decoration, on the other hand, was never encumbered by such pervasive practical restrictions for the simple reason that hair – at least the 'crowning glory' on our heads – seems to exist and to have evolved purely as a decorative and symbolic medium. Although it has been suggested that our ancestors retained and then extended the fur on the top of their heads as insulation against extremes of temperature, the lack of any correlation between hair length and climate undermines such thinking. Desmond Morris, in *Bodywatching*, proposes that our head hair developed originally as a species marker. As he points out, many primate species have distinctive patterns of head and facial hair that serve this purpose. This is a valid point but while Morris presumes a great stretch of time before we were 'sufficiently advanced, technologically to attack [hair] with knives and scissors [so as to] set about curtailing it in a thousand ways', it seems more likely that from the very start – and very probably coincidental with the gradual lengthening of head hair – our ancestors were finding ways of transforming natural hair into cultural artefacts. This presumption is based firstly on the universality of hair decoration in every known human society and, secondly, on the fact that without benefit of scissors or knives or other metal implements – often using only the most primitive of tools

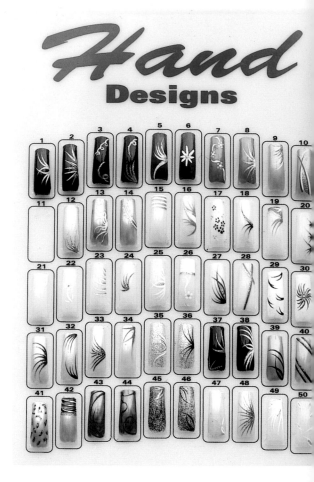

AIRBRUSHED AND ACRYLIC DESIGNS
offer an unlimited range of mini-masterpieces. Choice of nail colour is no longer determined by fashion trends but a matter of individual taste. Anything is possible. *above* airbrushed nail designs; *opposite* Lise shows off her own distinctive look in nail art and jewelry

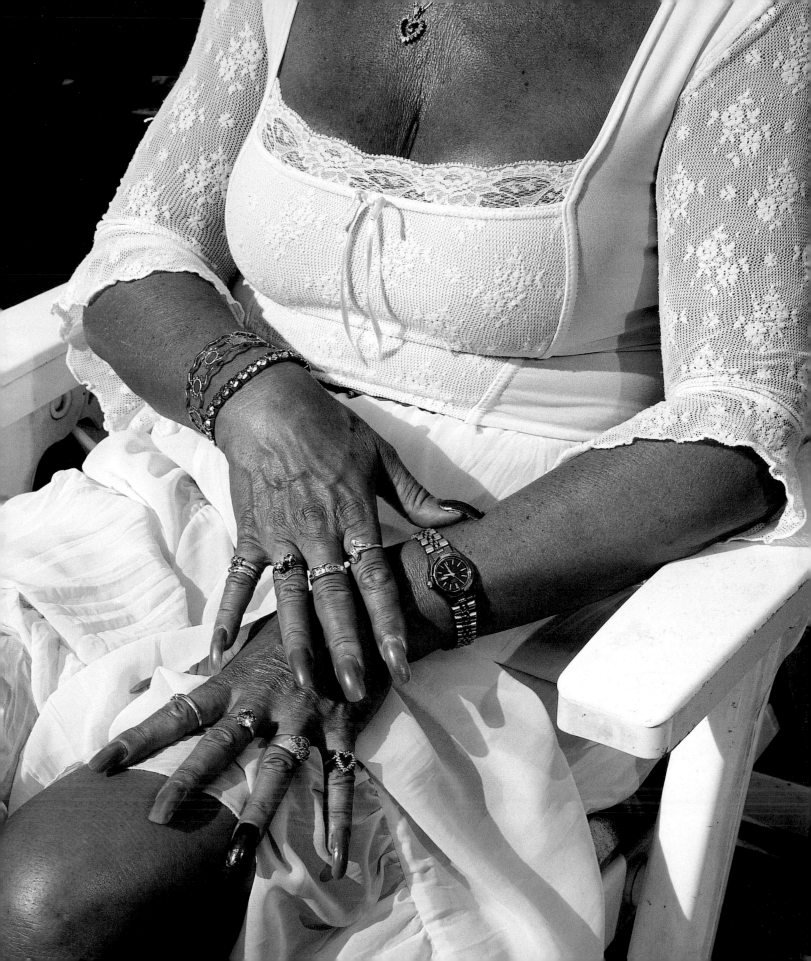

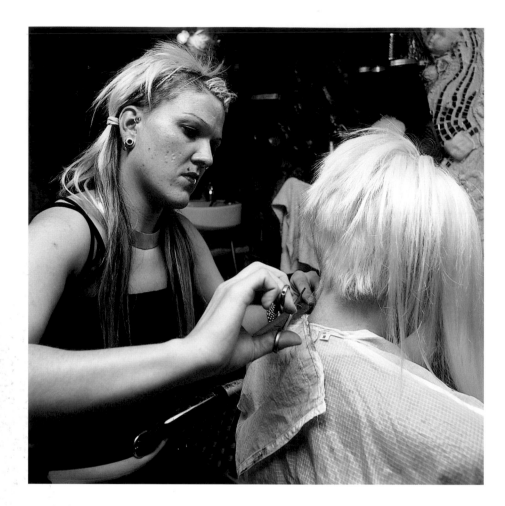

– tribal peoples have created hairstyles of such artistry and complexity as to make Marie Antoinette or any exotically coiffured fashion model seem banal in comparison. Morris is indeed right that our head hair serves as a species marker but what our 'crowning glory' is actually delineating is our species' unique capacity for transforming the body into an artistic, symbolic, cultural artefact – with each culture (and now, increasingly, each individual) transforming head hair in radically different ways. To this end we as a species have devised the most extraordinary range of techniques for transforming hair – a range of techniques unequalled by those for any other part of the body.

No doubt throughout most of human (pre)history hair was cut using tools made of stone, shell, bone or antler. The process was presumably uncomfortable and the results imprecise, but even with such implements, a wide range of distinctive styles would have been possible. Surprisingly, when metal tools such as knives (and later, scissors) became available, precision cutting was still rarely if ever critical to styling the hair. In Mary Trasko's view, in *Daring Do's:*

PRECISION CUTTING
lies at the heart of many contemporary hairstyles –
the creation of sharp, graphic styles with a focus not
just on the style but also on the quality of cut. Good
news for hairdressers. *opposite* getting a haircut at
Pepi's Hairspace; *below* Ane, Mock-Tudor hairstyle

A History of Extraordinary Hair, 'When the "bob" swept Europe and America
[from about 1913] the art of hairdressing centred for the first time on the
quality of the cut rather than the artifice of style.' As with most radically different styles of hair cutting, the bob was heavily laden with signification – in this
case, the emancipation of women. In the 1960s it would be longer styles for
men that challenged the status quo, as billboards proclaimed 'Make America
Beautiful – Get a Haircut!'. Whereas, previously, short crew cuts and flat-tops
(the front prodded up with a wax stick) seemed Modernist (for example that
of jazz musician Gerry Mulligan in the 1950s), next a short crop signified

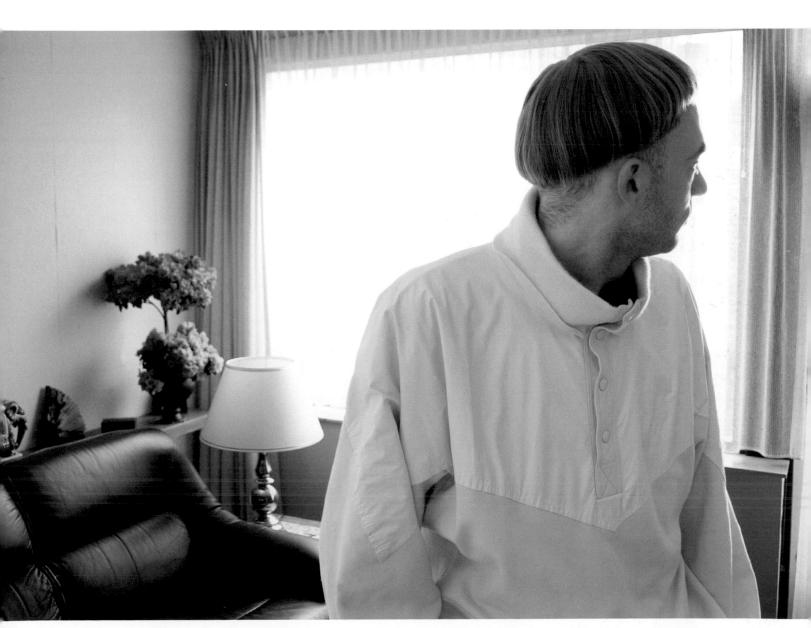

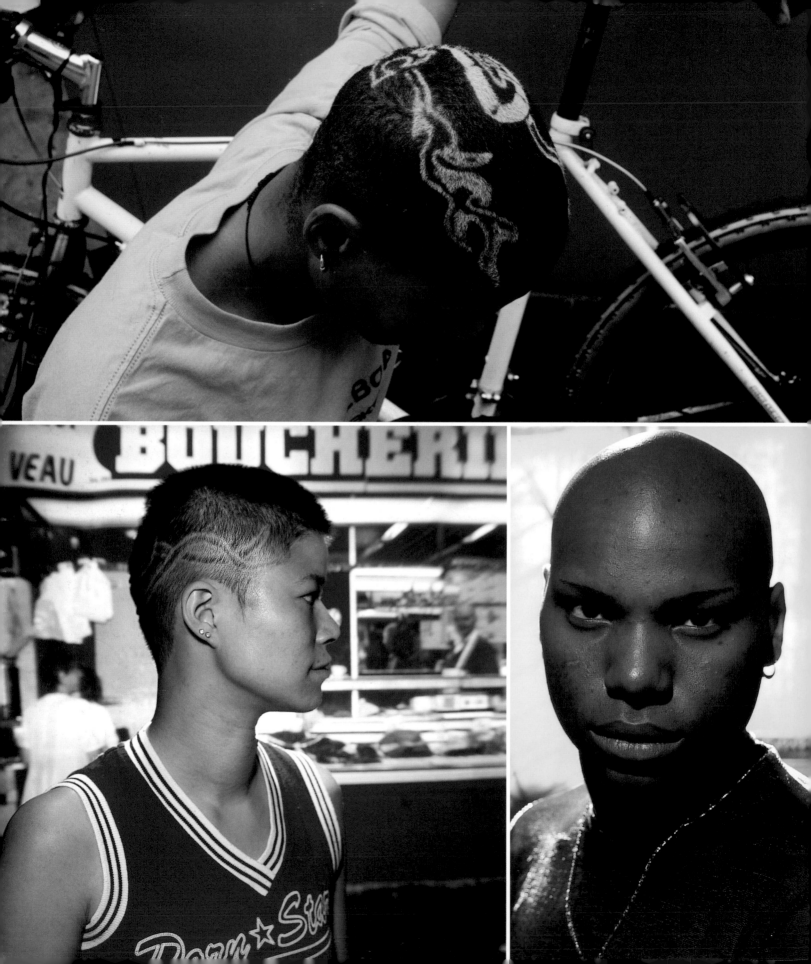

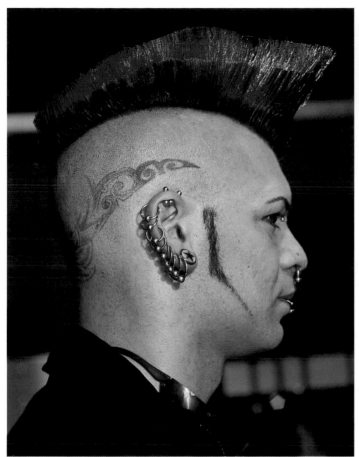 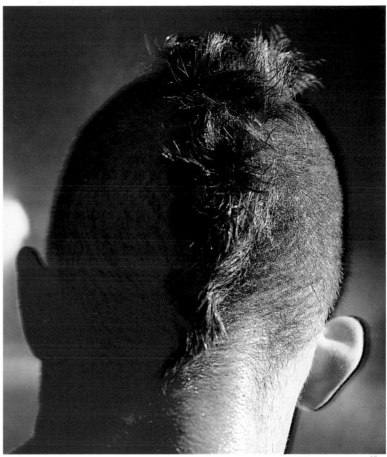

conformity, then racism (with the Skinheads in the late 1960s) and – confusing for many – homosexuality *à la* Gay Clone look of the 1970s.

The number of tribal peoples throughout the world who shave all or part of their heads (and did so prior to contact with the West) suggests great antiquity for this technique. Ditto hair plucking – for example using clam shells as tweezers. Most famous today is the Punks' Mohawk style, which featured shaved sides surrounding a central crest of long hair. This look was actually found among the Huron, Omaha and Osage tribes of the Great Plains. Among Amazonian peoples, a common style is a sort of reverse Mohawk in which a strip along the centre, rather than the sides, is shaved. Nuba men of the Sudan sometimes shave amazingly intricate designs into their tightly cropped hair – a style popular in our culture among hip hop musicians. Catholic monks and nuns in the Middle Ages shaved a round tonsure patch on the crown of their heads – a look shared with the Yanomamo of Venezuela. Head shaving often signifies an important rite of passage (as in the case of a young Masai warrior

SHAVING OR CLOSE-CROPPING
part or all of the scalp is an ancient form of hairstyling that has been revived to interesting effect by a wide range of subcultures. *opposite from top, clockwise* Ronald, close-cropped hair allows for further, graphic decoration using bleach and dye; Sonny, shaved eyebrows and head; Jenni-Li , patterns shaved into her hair by an Antillian barber; *above* Mauro, Mohawk and distinctive sideburns; *above right* Buddy, with Mohawk

who enters into the responsibilities of adulthood when his long, lion-like mane is shaved by his mother). Arguably, the most striking hairstyles of recent years have been those involving partial or complete shaving of women's scalps – a look first introduced by Punks, Goths and Modern Primitives.

Traditional peoples use a surprising range of substances as fixatives – including beeswax, clay, animal fats, butter, acacia gum, coconut oil, palm-kernel grease and honey – to hold hair in place and to sculpt it into extraordinary shapes. One of the most striking of such creations is the *boro* style worn by Hamar men of Ethiopia when they have been successful in war or hunting: brightly coloured clay is plastered over cropped hair in a sharp-edged, circular skullcap shape. Embedded in this clay is a macramé holder into which feathers are inserted. In Europe up until the 19th century, the standard hair fixative was gum paste. When this was replaced with a lard-based pomade, more OTT styles became possible. The introduction of new pomades for men (such as Brylcreem and NuNile) before World War II made possible the sculpted shapes of the D.A. (Duck's Ass) and the quiff (the greaser style of Tony Curtis and Elvis, which would be challenged by the Beatles' more natural look). Hairspray enabled a similar revolution to take place in women's styling around the same time – resulting in the bouffant, the towering beehive and, in the 1980s, Big Hair. To get their hair to defy gravity, the Punks used anything they could find: glue, KY Jelly, sugar, lard, toothpaste, washing-up liquid, margarine, butter, soap, egg whites and lemon juice. When Punk-influenced styles entered the mainstream in the 1980s, a new range of robust, sculptural fixatives became available.

Braiding, or plaiting as it is sometimes called, is a technique in which three or more sections of hair are woven together. It is found throughout the world and is a style of great antiquity – the regular, bumpy patterns on the heads of various Venus figures (the oldest surviving three-dimensional art) apparently show this style. Traditional Africa in particular is a rich source of wonderfully complex creations using this technique – especially cornrowing, which involves braiding tight to the scalp to produce intricate patterns. African slaves brought cornrowing to the New World but it was often derided and (except in the case of young girls) virtually disappeared. In America in the 1970s, however, following on from the success of the 'Black Is Beautiful' Afro (ironically, a style far too naturalistic for most people in Africa), braided styles enjoyed (and

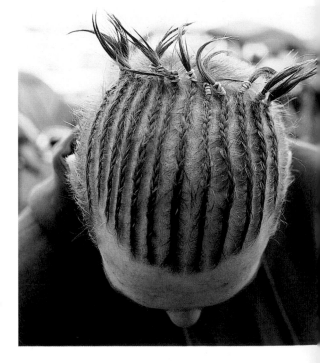

BRAIDING OR PLAITING WEAVES OR KNOTS
three or more strands of hair together. From African roots, it is now part of global culture. Cornrowing uses braiding tight to the scalp to produce intricate patterns of contrasting hair and skin. *above* a French biker with intricate cornrowing; *opposite, clockwise from left* Ghyslaine at Emm & Bee's, also with cornrowing, in black hair; Karen, UK, extensions braided into her hair by Ghyslaine; Irina, Finland, with long blonde braids

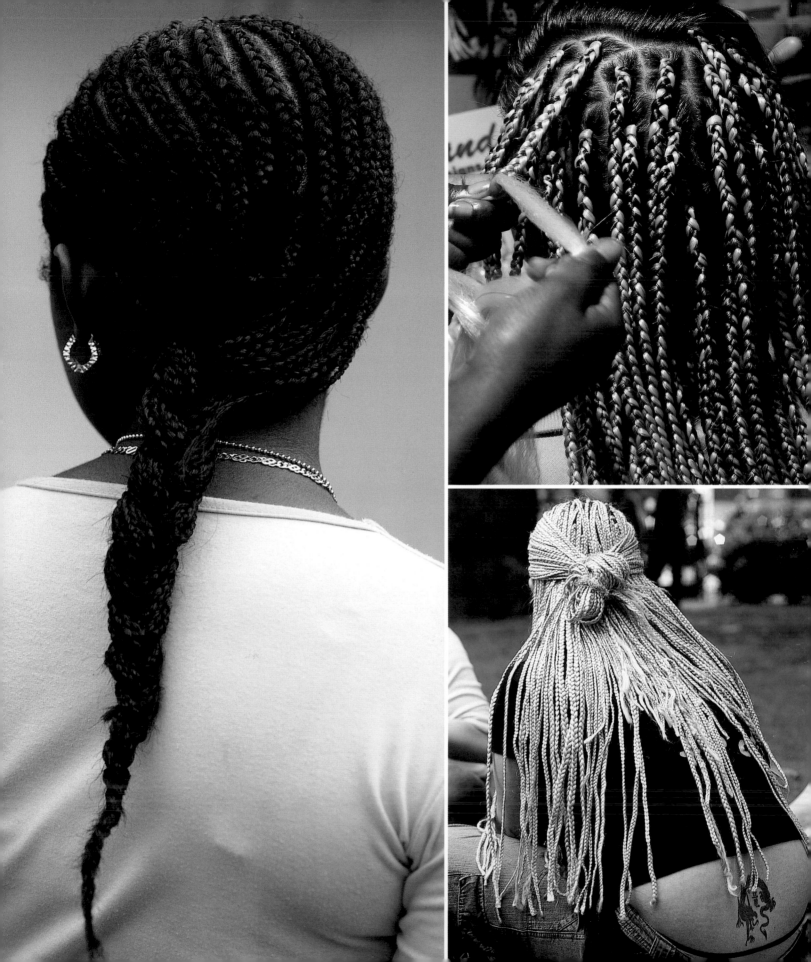

continue to enjoy) enormous popularity. Although this has prompted many would-be street cred non-blacks to imitate it, intricate, tightly braided styles are most successful on Negroid hair. Looser forms of braiding work well on all types of hair – as can be seen in one of the most famous hairstyles of the 1990s, that of Lara Croft.

A wide range of objects and materials has been used to shape and support the hair, throughout the world and throughout history; most simply, string or ribbon to tie clumps of hair into ponytails or, in Japan, the distinctive topknots – *chonmage* – sported by Samurai warriors and sumo wrestlers. The pigtails or queues that were once a symbol of China were banned in 1912 post-revolution because of their associations with the old rulers. Simple headbands were once common among Australian Aborigines and some North American Indians (presumably the inspiration for the headbands of Hippies in the 1960s). The threading styles found in various parts of Africa – and now extremely popular with Afro-Americans – take the simple process of winding black thread around sectioned hair to achieve mind-boggling results: spiky, radiating antennae or interlocking strands of hair architecture. Throughout much of European history, hairnets (favoured also by the Big Men of New Guinea), hairpins and combs served either to keep hair in place or to allow it to be piled high on top of the head in seemingly precarious constructions. Even more flamboyant, gravity-defying creations have been achieved with the use of cylinder-shaped metal frames (Mangbetu women of Central Africa); bamboo hoops that surround the head like a halo, and to which sections of hair are attached (women in Zaire); and the huge wire, horsehair and wool padded frames that made possible the towering *têtes* worn by aristocratic French women prior to the Revolution – structures so tall that women had to crouch on the floors of their carriages and (at least in the cartoonists' caricatures) hairdressers were required to mount ladders and swing from scaffolding. (And which, especially as hair was adhered to these structures with lashings of lard, unfortunately provided cosy homes for mice and other vermin.)

Natural hair colour is determined by the number and shape of melanin granules in hair cells: a lot of elongated granules producing black hair, fewer producing blonde and the presence of spherical or oval shaped granules resulting in a reddish hue. As with every other feature of appearance, human beings have rarely been content with what nature gives them and have used colouring

ADDING OBJECTS TO THE HAIR,
either as ornament or to shape it, is an ancient practice that can produce looks that are contemporary and fresh. *opposite* Vianney with hair tied up in a side ponytail; *opposite right* Giovanca with red extensions and flowers

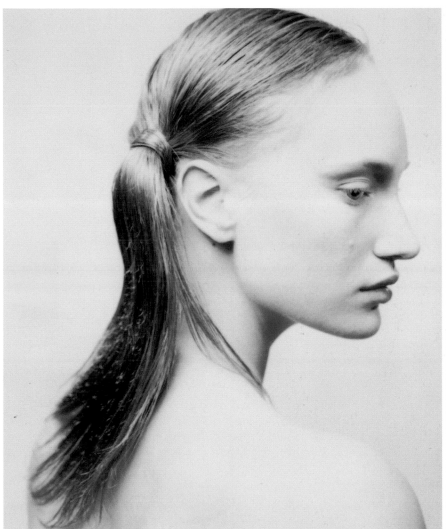
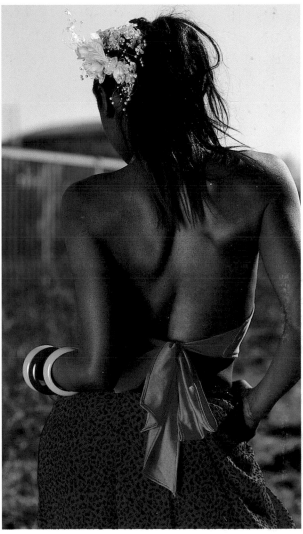

and beaching to change their hair – often with truly astounding results. For example the Indians of the Xingu National Park in the Amazon have long made a particularly vivid, fire-engine-red paste from the seeds of the urucu plant. Using a piece of string, this is smeared over pudding-basin haircuts, which may be further enlivened by painting jet-black designs on top of the red. Elsewhere, as well as plant extracts, minerals provide a source of vivid hair colourant. As well as their body painting, the men of the Nuba of the Sudan are renowned for their closely cropped, yellow, red, blue and orange hair. Henna is used in many parts of the world to darken hair; everything from apricot kernels to a mixture of ash and cow urine to lighten it. Both the ancient Greeks and Romans were keen on lightening their hair, but often with disastrous results: as Ovid commented to his mistress, 'Didn't I tell you, "cease to dye your hair"? And now you

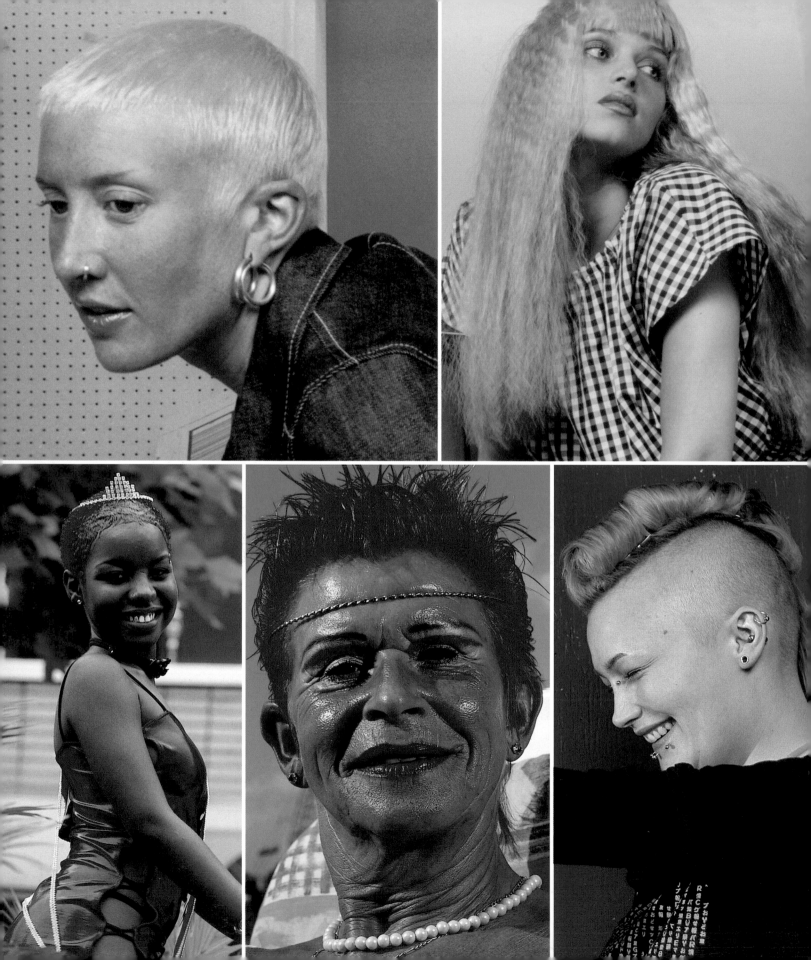

THE EASE AND SCOPE FOR CHANGING HAIR

colour and style has increased through technological advances. Humans have long used bleaches, dyes and pigments but, in the West, it was the Punks who opened the creative floodgates. *opposite from top left, clockwise* Kirsten with bleached, cropped hair; Marina, with crimped hair; Anja; Lise; a Carnival princess, have all used permanent dye

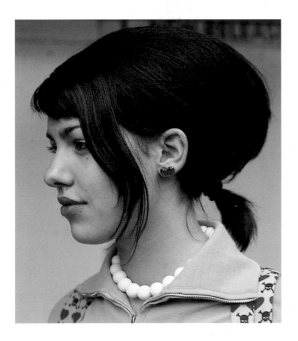

TEASING OR BACKCOMBING,

once called frizzing, dramatically increases the volume of hair and allows new shapes to be created. *above* Alina, with a contemporary take on 1950s bouffant style

have no hair to dye'. More successful – albeit not long-lasting – were the powders (sometimes in blue, violet, pink and yellow as well as 'natural' shades) that were blown over hair (or wigs) in the 17th and 18th centuries. Peroxide for bleaching the hair was introduced in the 1920s. When this became the first step of a two-part process involving methyl violet or methylene blue the result was the platinum blonde shade, which looked fantastic on the silver screen. The home-hair-dyeing kits that were introduced in the 1950s with provocative advertising campaigns – 'Does she or doesn't she?'; 'Blondes have more fun' – made changing the colour of your hair (at least for women) a normal occurrence. But, leaving Jean Harlow and Marilyn Monroe behind, the trend moved increasingly towards shades that might look natural. It was left to David Bowie's Ziggy Stardust and then, in the late 1970s, the Punks' exuberance for Krazy Kolor, to bring hair colouring back to that delight in artifice found among tribal peoples.

Combs discovered in the Indus valley date from four thousand five hundred years ago, but implements for dividing and untangling the hair likely existed long before. In an age when plastic combs can be manufactured quickly and cheaply, it is easy to forget what an achievement of technology and craftsmanship it must have been to carve out the long delicate teeth of the first such tools. As well as untangling hair, combs have been used throughout history to help to keep hair in place and as ornaments. Interestingly, the use of the comb really came into its own as a technique for styling hair when it was used to deliberately entangle it. The fashion for frizzing (what is today called backcombing or teasing) began in France in 1550 and was desirable because it provided enough volume for covering wire frames and pads. The practice caught on again some four hundred years later when a combination of curlers, hooded driers, stronger hairsprays and frantic backcombing resulted in the bouffant and the ultimate achievement of the hair-hoppers (particularly enthusiastic backcombers), the beehive – a look that is know as Chicken Beak in the Kingdom of Benin, where high hair is equated with social status.

While the West has seen a bewildering range of hairstyles come and go (and, more often than not, come back into fashion again) the comb and brush have remained key implements for hairstyling. Indeed, throughout most of Western history, combing or brushing the hair has been synonymous with being well groomed and even with being of good character, respectable. Perhaps for this

DREADLOCKS REQUIRE THAT HAIR
be left uncombed, unlike most hairstyles today.
Undoubtedly extremely ancient, dreadlocked hair
came to be associated in the previous century with
Bob Marley and other Rastafarians; in the 21st century
it is an enduring style for black hair and seen throughout
Western culture. Although most hair types will group
naturally into locks, most desired dread styles require
a great deal of care and attention. *clockwise from
right* Daryl, USA; Sharon, Netherlands; Sherwin,
Trinidad; Sam, Cameroon

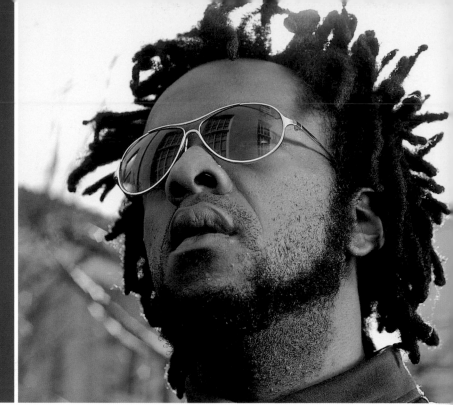

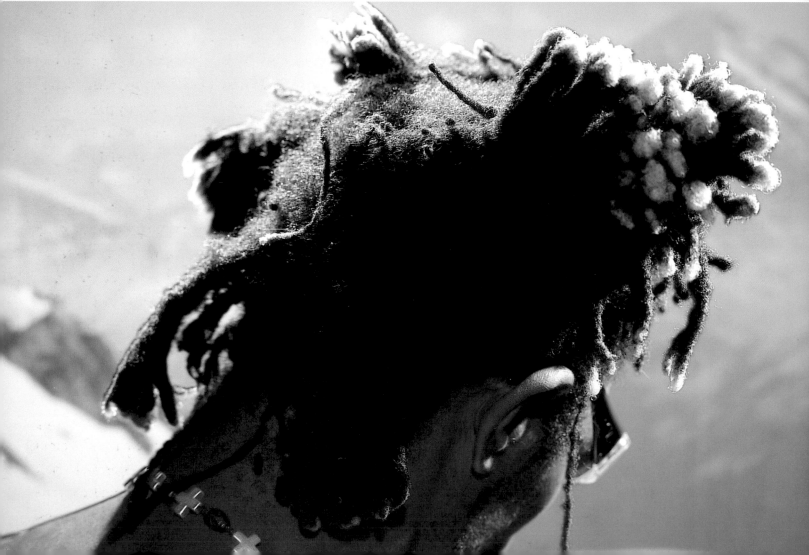

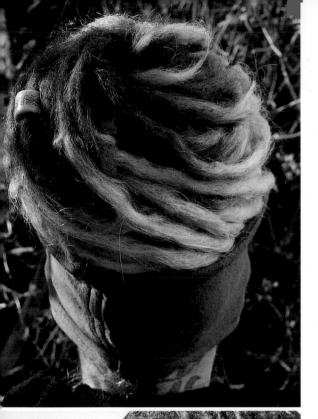

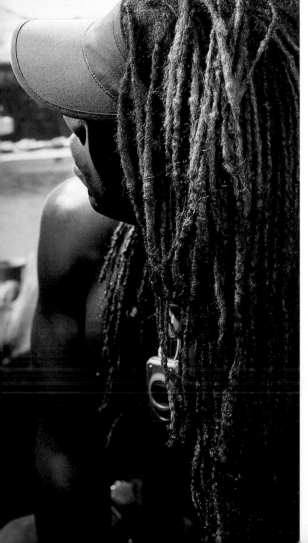

reason, the dreadlocks worn by Bob Marley and other Rastafarians (originally from Jamaica but now spread across the world) were often criticized as 'unkempt'. In truth, however, the twisting of segments of hair into locks is an alternative (and, clearly, extremely ancient) approach to haircare and styling. Although many types of hair (in particular but not only black) would naturally form into locks if nothing was done to it, regular and persistent grooming (washing, slow drying, oiling, separating out strands, etc.) is required to achieve the desired effect. Linked to Rastafarianism in the 20th century, dreadlocks (largely through their association with reggae music) have come to be worn by many – including Caucasians – who are not followers of this religion. However, even if worn simply as fashion, in standing outside and thereby opposing hundreds if not thousands of years during which the West came to equate respectability and even civilization itself with the act of combing or brushing the hair into individuals strands (think of Victorian novels in which the essential good character of the heroine is signalled by rigorous hair-brushing) dreadlocks can never be entirely devoid of a powerful symbolic significance – one that challenges an exclusively Western (and white) definition of civilization.

Some people like curly hair, some straight hair. Unfortunately people aren't always born with the kind of hair they desire. Various curling and straightening techniques have been employed, with varying degrees of success. The ancient Egyptians wound hair around rods and then coated it with beeswax. The Assyrians found this worked better if the rods were heated. The Victorians – who believed curly locks belied a sweet temperament – went crazy about the 'ondulations' made by a process involving curlers and heated irons invented by the Frenchman Marcel Grateau (often with the result of damaging their hair). The first permanent waving machine, which appeared in 1906, used a combination of temperature and chemistry. Expensive, taking as long as twelve hours, it also often destroyed the hair it was supposed to make beautifully curly. In the 1940s a cold perm method opened the door to safe home perming. The conk (also known as fixed or relaxed hair) began in the 1920s among Afro-Americans who yearned for straight rather than tightly curled hair. Involving lye and a hot comb, the process was painful and often damaging to the hair. In his 1965 autobiography Malcolm X (himself conked in his youth) argued that it was also psychologically and politically dangerous, as it was founded on the presumption that blacks could only be beautiful by imitating Caucasians.

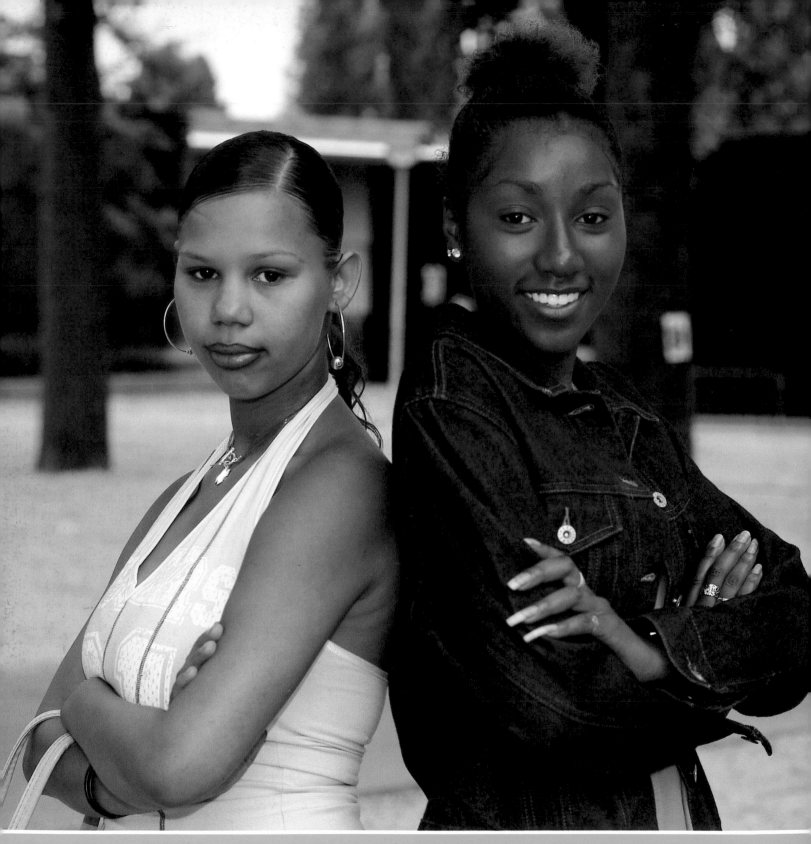

MAKING CURLY HAIR STRAIGHT
(or 'relaxed', as it is sometimes called) or straight hair curly, there is seemingly
no end to how hair can be transformed – colour, volume, texture and shape.
above Stephanie and Mignella with black lip liner, false nails and relaxed hair;
opposite girls at Carnival, Rotterdam, with curled hair extensions added to Afro hair

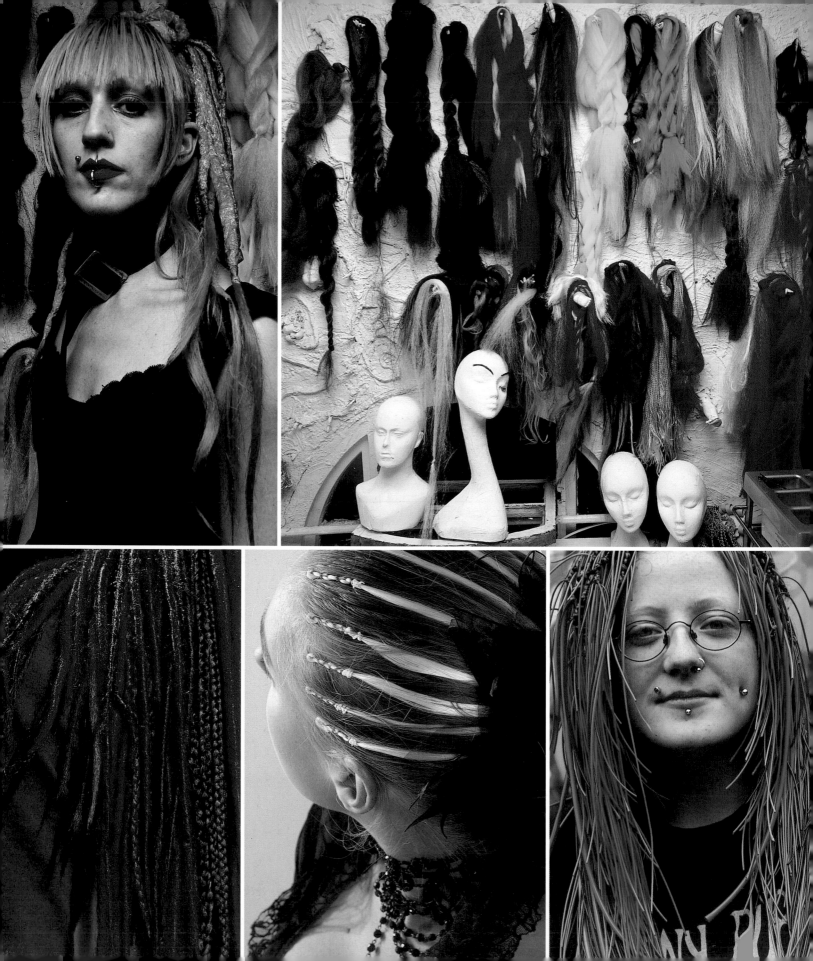

Subsequently the relaxed hair worn by most black musicians came to be seen as politically incorrect. More recently, however, this view has been challenged by female hip hop artists who have argued that processed hair and black pride can coexist comfortably.

Hairpieces and extensions have a long history as techniques for transforming the appearance of hair. Many traditional peoples use their own or a relative's hair clippings to give greater length or bulk to their coiffure. In many parts of Africa sisal fibres serve the same purpose. Whatever material is used, methods such as braiding and threading allow extensions to be attached easily. If the clippings used have been treated chemically, then more dramatic effects can be achieved with colour. Hairpieces were used extensively by Victorian and Edwardian women who appreciated the additional volume. They were also popular in the 1950s and 1960s because they allowed Western women to keep up with ever-accelerating fashion changes. In the 1990s the Spanish-born but London-based team at Pepi's took hairstyling to new dimensions when they invented a technique for using fluorescent plastic tubing as futuristic hair extensions.

Taking the attachment of hair further is the wig. Some of the most elaborate and extraordinary wigs come from traditional societies. In particular, in the highlands of New Guinea – where the ghosts of ancestors are believed to reside in the hair, and baldness or thinning hair indicates that these spirits have abandoned a man – men wear enormous wigs made of carefully collected hair clippings supported by a huge frame, brightly painted and decorated with scarab beetles, feathers and fur. Usually a man will make his own wig (a task too important to entrust to others) and to ensure its brightness and power he will not have sex during its construction. Both men and women wore wigs in ancient Egypt: made from human hair, wool, cotton and palm-leaf fibre (even pure silver in one instance), these were stiffened with beeswax and sometimes dyed red, green or blue. In ancient Rome prostitutes were obliged to wear blonde wigs. When Messalina (wife of Emperor Claudius) mischievously wore one, they became a fashion. (Luckily, Rome's northern conquests supplied plenty of blonde hair.)

The early Christian church was opposed to wig wearing, arguing that a blessing from God, through the touch of the priest's hand on the head, couldn't be transmitted through someone else's hair (which, just as alarmingly, might

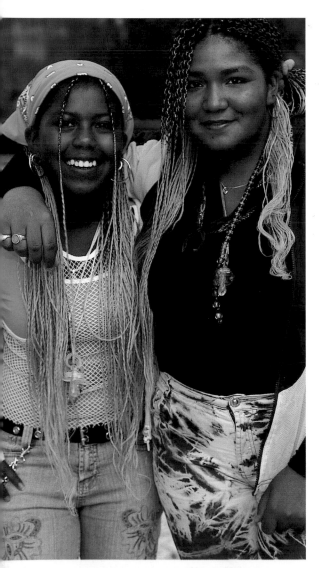

FROM NATURAL HAIR TO FLUORESCENT plastic cable, the length of hair can now be extended with a variety of materials. In the process, colour and texture can also be altered. *opposite from top left, clockwise* Pepi's Hairspace, brightly dyed hair extensions; synthetic hair extensions in every imaginable colour; Michelle, with plastic cable extensions and multiple facial piercings; Goth Denise with elaborate hair extensions plaited in; Hannu with purple extensions; *above* Marilva and Janice

have come from a damned or unclean person). As is so often the case in matters of appearance, this had little if any impact. The great era of Western wig wearing came in the 17th and 18th centuries when everyone (even labourers and farmers) wore wigs. At least initially it was men in particular who favoured this decoration, and their enormous styles give us the expression 'bigwig' (which could equally be used to describe the men of New Guinea). Given the complicated, time-consuming hairstyles of the time – and the infrequency of washing – wigs were actually both convenient and hygienic. Queen Elizabeth I had some eighty different wigs in a wide range of colours. Each profession had its own style. The Victorians, however, were less keen on wigs (eventually retaining them only for lawyers and judges) and it was only in the 1960s, with the introduction of fun wigs made of synthetic hair, that wig wearing won back some of its popularity. By allowing the wearer to change personalities in an instant and experiment with the most exotic looks, such transformations (as they are sometimes termed by Afro-Americans) continue to catch the eye at parties, in clubs and in pop videos. Less visible but at least as numerous are the necessity wigs that are worn to cover baldness. Although wigmakers have made such 'rugs' ever more realistic, more and more Western men are turning to transplants, during which individual hair follicles are moved from one part of the scalp to another.

As well as long hair sprouting from the tops of their heads, human beings also have patches of shorter, fur-like hair on the face and body. The presence and extent of this hair varies with race, gender and individual predisposition. As with head hair, human beings often remove or modify this body hair rather than simply leaving such growth to take its natural course.

Eyebrows and eyelashes are present in all races and both genders. They serve obvious practical functions protecting the eyes (and, at least as importantly, in non-verbal communication), yet they are also often a focus of adornment. Eyebrows are or were shaved or plucked in many traditional societies; the same was true of women in medieval Europe. In the 20th century many women followed the Hollywood fashion for removing the natural eyebrows and then painting in new ones. Eyelashes are also plucked out in some traditional societies, whereas in the West, at least for women, a wide range of techniques has been employed to make them more prominent. Artificial lashes first became popular in the 1940s, when waterproof mascara and eyelash curlers were also

FUN WIGS OFFER AN INSTANT NEW IDENTITY for parties, special events and music videos, loudly proclaiming their artifice in every style and colour. Having fallen out of favour with the Victorians, except for certain professional duties such as presiding in court, ostentatious wig-wearing for men and women has been rejuvenated by fun wigs. *below* R. Smith, wearing lilac wig and glasses; *opposite* wigs and body painting worn as a stunt to advertise a radio station

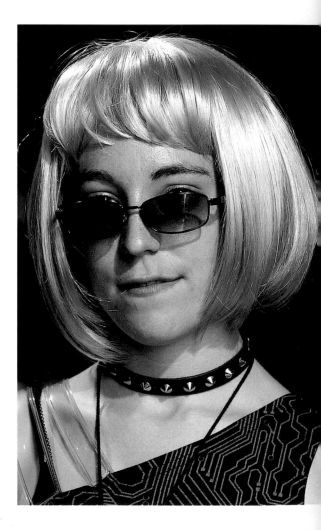

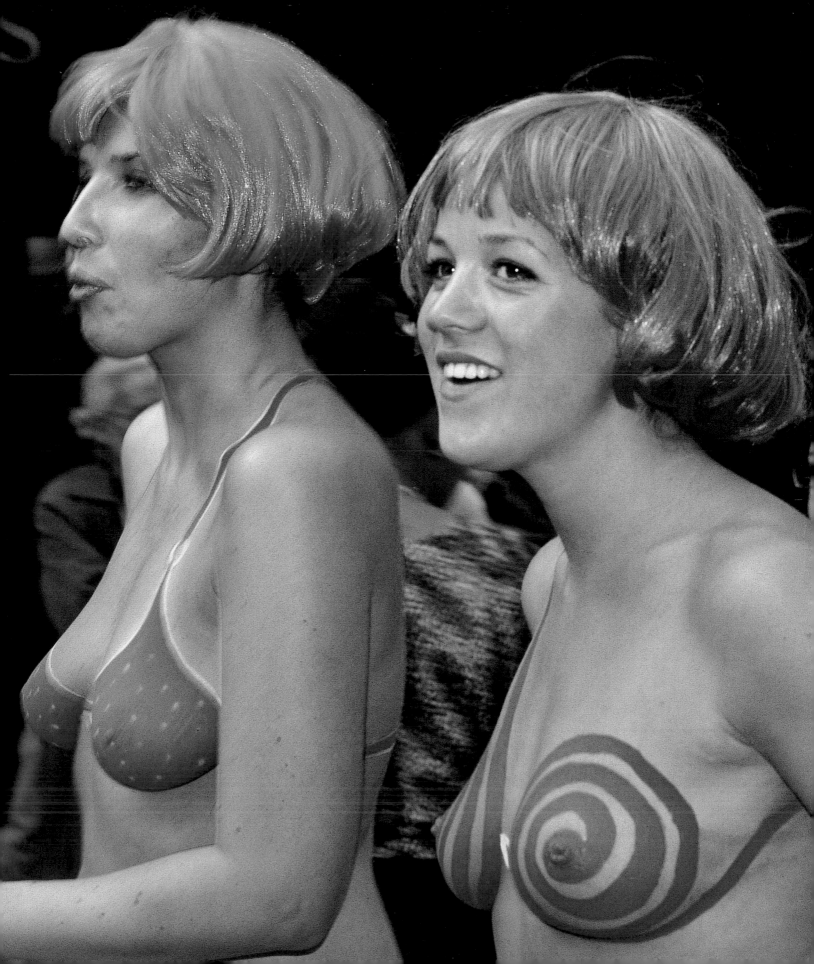

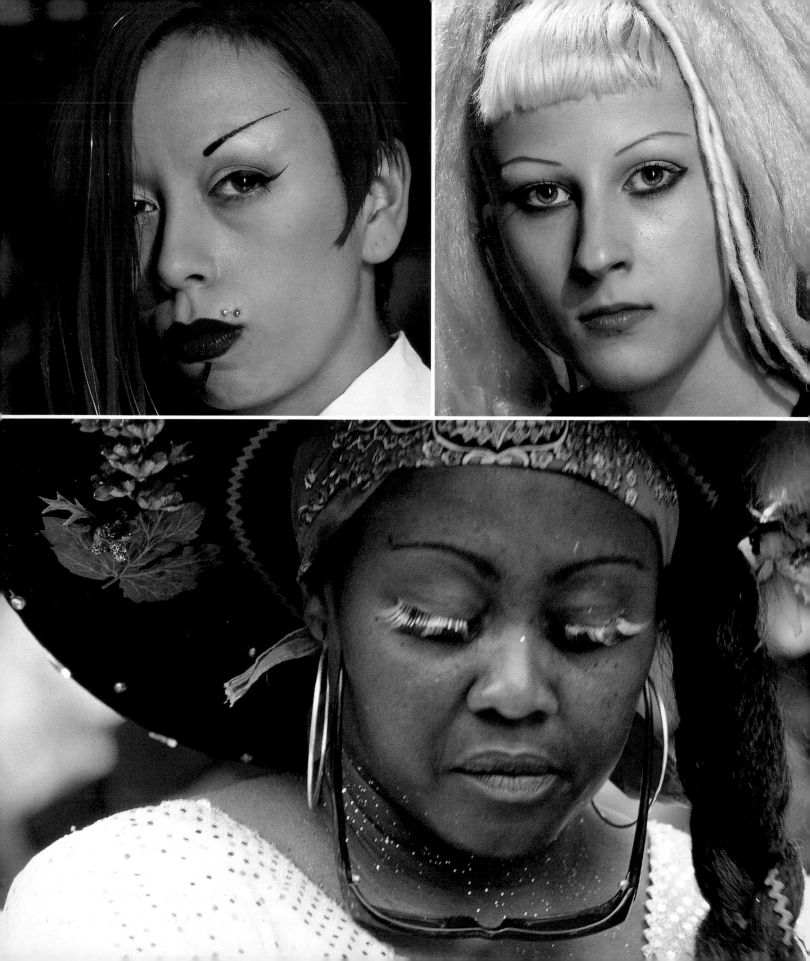

EYEBROWS AND EYELASHES

help to protect the eyes but are also vitally important in non-verbal communication. Modifying or removing them offers yet another technique for transforming appearance. Eyebrows are trimmed, plucked, or shaved and replaced with painted, stylized versions; eyelashes often visually accentuated with paint or extensions. *opposite from top left, clockwise* Sarah, manager at clothing shop Cyberdog, with shaved and repainted eyebrows; Veronica, also with painted eyebrows; fake foil eyelashes at Carnival, Rotterdam; *below* Nicola, with shaved and repainted eyebrows

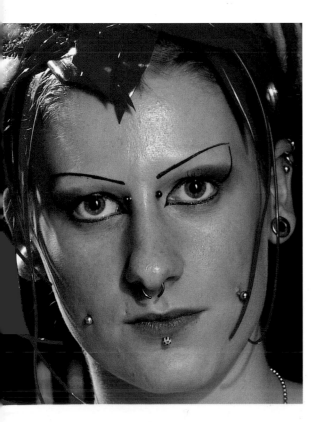

introduced. The 1960s saw huge painted-on eyelashes, false lashes produced in rows (including some made of foil and glitter) and more startling colours of mascara. In the 21st century, having an eyelash perm is now common practice for Japanese women.

Hair elsewhere on the face is much more likely in males and clearly developed as a gender marker. Although men in a few traditional societies actively cultivate their facial growth (in the New Guinea highlands men paint and decorate their big beards with leaves), shaving or plucking is surprisingly common. Western history has seen innumerable pendulum swings between hairy and clean-faced ideals: the ancient Egyptian nobility was clean-shaven but wore false beards (including women); in Greece the nobility was bearded; most Romans were scrupulously clean-shaven (using the first shaving creams and straight razors) whereas the barbarians who invaded Rome, as their name suggests, were the bearded ones. Subject to fashion, male facial growth has also long been the focus of religious doctrine, though never consensus — in some instances free-flowing beards being equated with spiritual attainment, in others just the opposite.

As with all other aspects of body decoration, facial hair growth is no longer — for the first time in human history — rigidly determined by social background, occupation or fashion trends. Men now have unprecedented freedom in these matters and (perhaps balancing women's greater freedom with cosmetics) have been experimenting in ever greater numbers. There are countless possibilities to choose from: the full beard, goatee, various moustaches, sideburns, designer stubble and the soul patch (small area of hair under the lower lip) plus various combinations thereof. Whatever design is chosen, it inevitably reverberates with meaning. From God to Satan, Santa Claus to Hitler, Abe Lincoln to Osama bin Laden, every style of beard has powerful historical and semiological associations. Indeed, facial hair constitutes one of our most extensive and powerful visual language systems.

While body hair is typically more abundant in human males than females, it is found in both sexes. In particular, it grows under the armpits and at the crotch where there are also very high concentrations of scent-producing glands — the hair helping with odour production and retention. Human beings are the most highly scented of all primates (see D. Michael Stoddart's fascinating book *The Scented Ape*). It is thought that while we have retained these glands and the

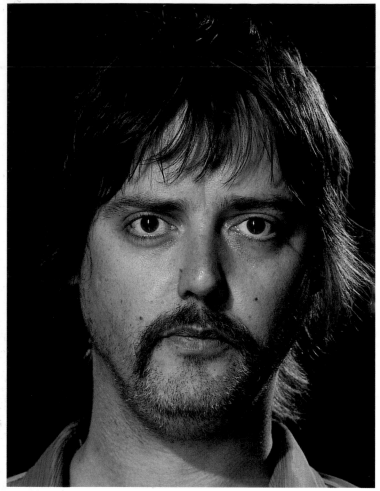

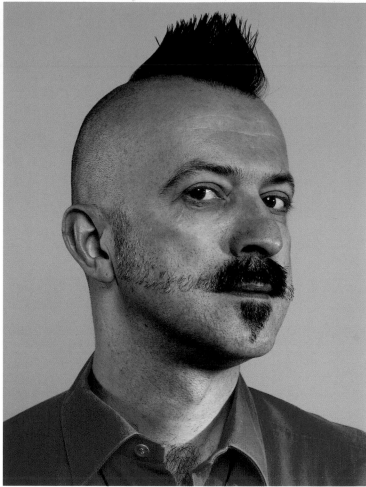

patches of hair that assist them, our ancestors, finding the sexual stimulation of these odours too disruptive of tribal life, gradually evolved negative rather than positive associations for these aromas. Enter deodorants and the removal of such hair.

The primary reason why we remove body hair is visual rather than olfactory. For some time it has been the norm in most Western societies for women to remove their underarm hair, but recent years have also seen a significant trend towards the trimming and often complete removal of women's pubic hair. Indeed, many if not most women (and a growing number of men) are coming to define all body hair as unwanted – with electrolysis and laser treatments joining depilatory creams, wax, razors and tweezers in the war against the horror of unsightly hair. Interestingly, a great many tribal peoples have exactly the same obsession – scraping, plucking and pumicing themselves to hairless perfection without the benefit of the latest triple-bladed razors. As the Nuba of the Sudan see it, the defining feature of our humanity is not language (which the Nuba believe monkeys also possess) but shaving.

TO SHAVE OR NOT TO SHAVE,
that is the question. And today there is no single, correct answer. Men have unprecedented freedom in choosing how to display – or remove – their facial hair. The result is an idiosyncratic vocabulary of beards, moustaches, sideburns and little tufts of hair under the lower lip called 'soul patches'. *above left* Glen, with '1970s porn-style' moustache; *above* jewelry designer and manager at Galerie Ra Paul Derrez, with manicured facial and head hair; *opposite* John, with full beard and moustache

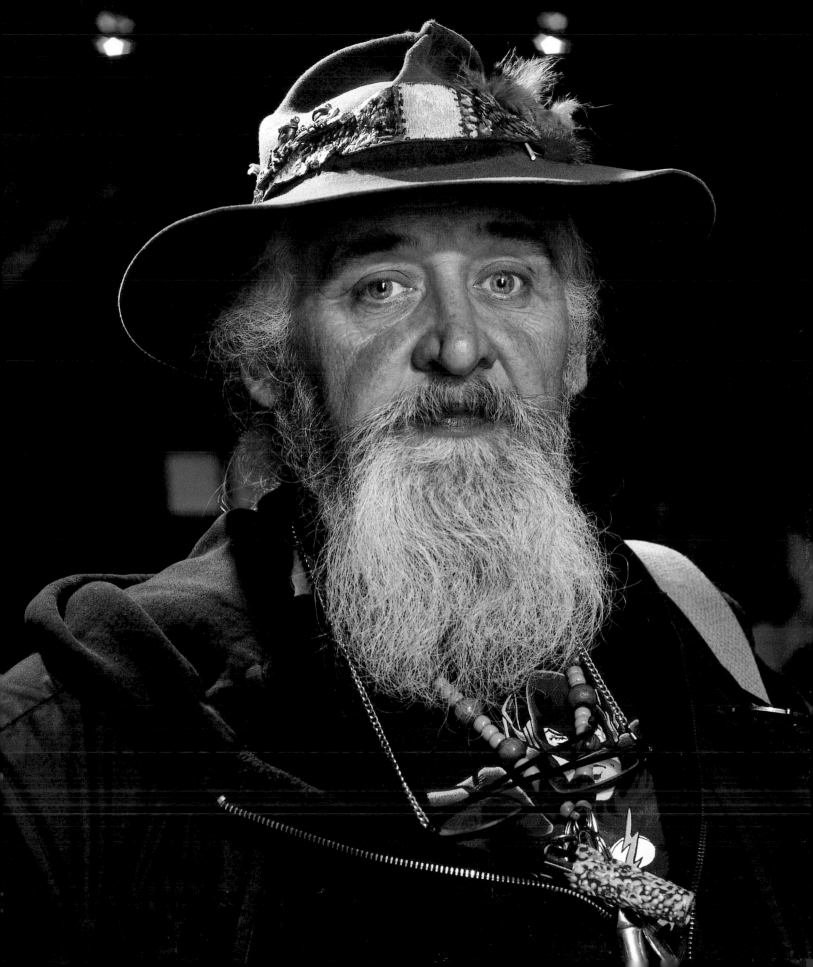

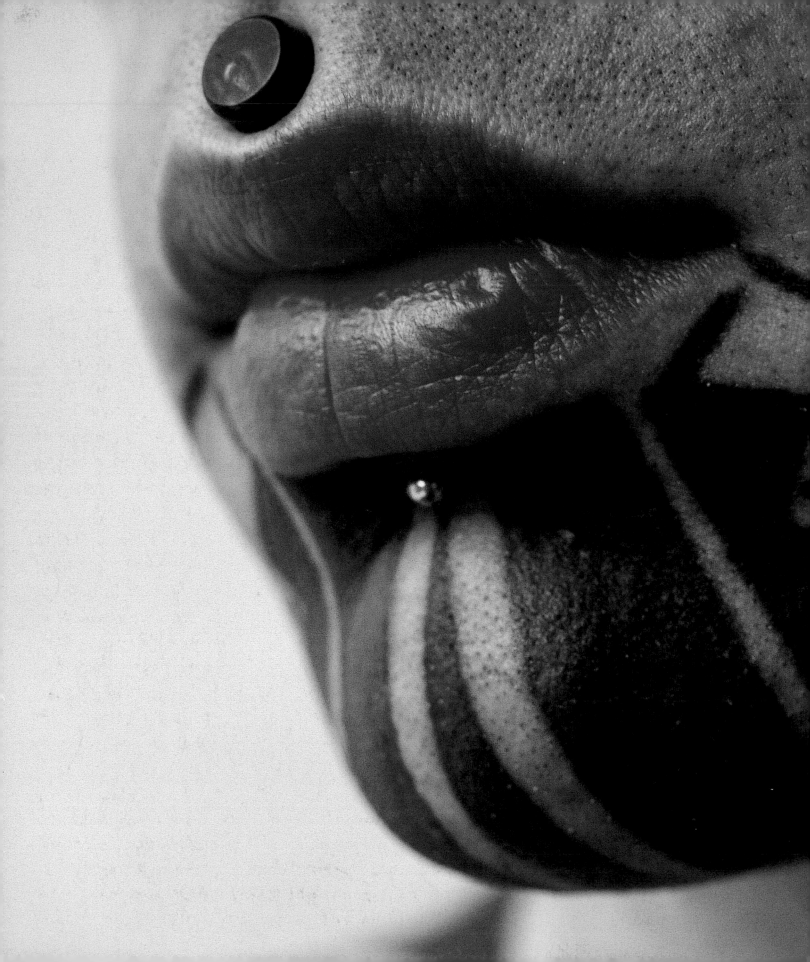

CHAPTER SIX

THE EXOTIC BODY

In any traditional society people decorate their bodies in the styles and using the techniques set down by their culture over countless generations. Indeed, the colours, design motifs and techniques that have come to be seen as beautiful and appropriate offer a remarkably succinct symbolic distillation of the values, beliefs and history of a particular people. In short, by transforming their appearance, traditional peoples themselves, in the styling and decoration of their bodies, become visual symbols – advertisements, so to speak – of their culture. And always, it is their own rather than someone else's culture that they proudly display.

In the Western world more often than not people delight in decorating their bodies with the styles and ornaments of other cultures: the Indian bracelet, the African hair braiding, the Tahitian-style tattoo, the eye make-up of Cleopatra (or, at least, Elizabeth Taylor), the henna design from Morocco, the Mohican razored hair favoured by the Punks, all manner of primitive piercings (even if some are actually of Western invention). Surely an intergalactic anthropologist coming to earth to study human culture would find this disinclination of the West towards its own indigenous styles of body decoration a bit strange? Why do Westerners apparently want to look like everyone but themselves? Is this a sign of alienation, estrangement from their own culture? Or could it be that this attraction to the exotic is simply an inevitable result of living at a time when exploration, trade and travel have brought them knowledge of so many different cultures and

THE EXOTIC INSPIRES DECORATION
in many forms. *these pages* Dave at Tusk,
moko-inspired chin tattoo and lip plug

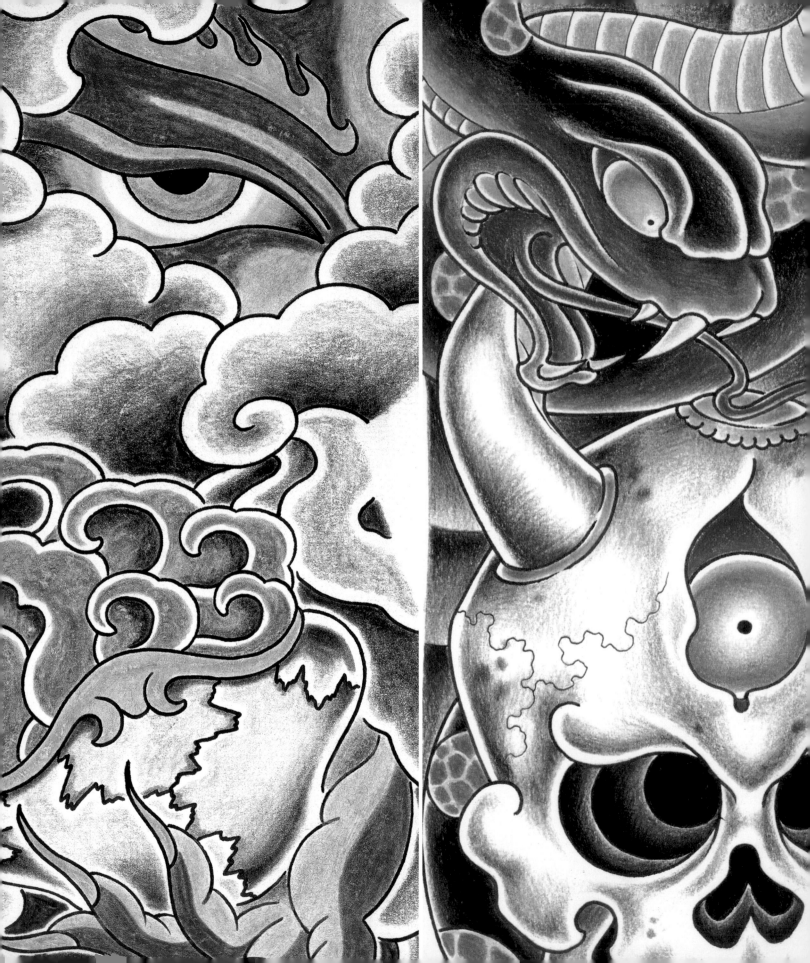

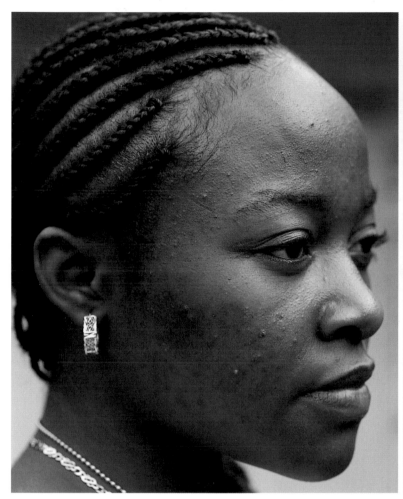

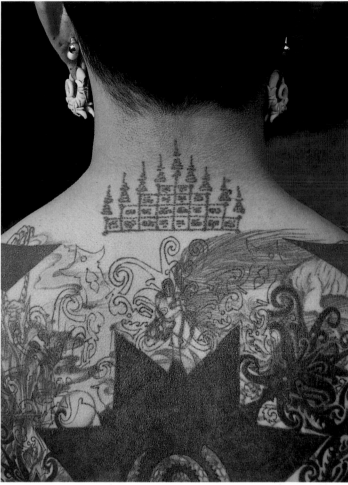

their different styles of body decoration (something an intergalactic anthropologist would surely know all about)?

It has often been said that *Playboy* was so successful because it celebrated 'the girl next door'. Perhaps, but often our desires seem most stimulated not by the cosy familiarity of the girl or boy next door, but rather by the exotic body. Thus Anthony fell for Cleopatra. Wealthy Englishmen travelled to Italy on the Grand Tour in the 18th and 19th centuries ostensibly in search of culture but, as guidebooks of the time make clear, the beauty of the Italian women was a persistent preoccupation. Gauguin set up his easel in Tahiti. 'Little Egypt' (aka American May Howard) stunned them with her belly dancing at the 1893 Chicago World's Fair. Paris went crazy for Josephine Baker.

Today, manga artists in modern Tokyo lust after their super-Westernized fantasy women while Japanese girls long for Western popstars. Throughout the world the tourist industry continues to cater to and be supported by the appeal

ABSORBING AND DELIGHTING IN EXOTIC influences, Western culture is affected today by the broadest geographic range of styles in its history. Often permanently applied directly to the body in the form of tattoos, piercings, jewelry, hairstyling, henna and make-up, Western body decoration is increasingly defined by the mix and persistence of other cultures. *opposite far left* tattoo design by Yorg at Medusa Tattoo, Athens and *opposite* tattoo design by Alex Binnie at Into You, London, both showing Tibetan influence; *above* Ghyslaine, hairdresser at Emm & Bee's, London, with African-style cornrowing; *above right* Marc, Australia, a mixture of Bornean-influenced tattoos and jewelry 'I live it and love it, and it is what we are trying to revive.'

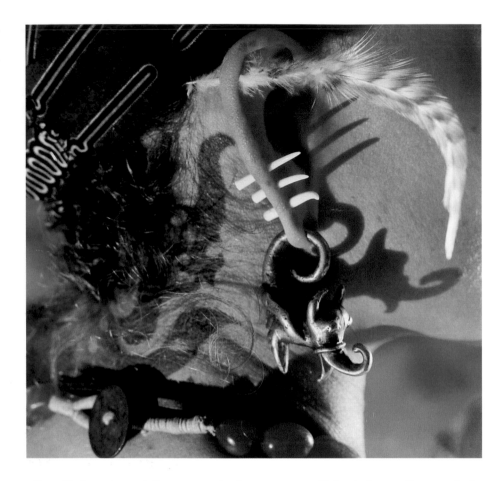

of exotic beauty and the prospect of romance on distant shores. Desperate to compete, the girl or boy next door employs all manner of body decoration techniques – cosmetics, hairstyling, henna, ornament, tanning or skin lightening, tattooing and piercing – in the hope of becoming the foreign, exotic other.

Western fashion has long been enriched and enlivened by the importation of all sorts of exotic styles, and this has been as evident in body decoration techniques as in clothing design – the Oriental, Arabian Nights and ancient Egyptian influences on, for example, Erté, Fortuny, Poiret and Saint Laurent each had their counterparts in cometics. Hollywood also benefited from the exotic appeal of many of its stars – for example, Pola Negri, Dolores Del Rio, Anna May Wong, Carmen Miranda – and even went so far as to take a young woman from Cincinnati, Ohio, and reinvent her as Sahara-desert-born Theda Bara, 'woman of mystic powers', to play the parts of Salome and Cleopatra.

While some male stars – such as Valentino 'The Sheik' – also benefited from their purported exoticism, such exoticism rarely impacted directly on male fashion except for the occasional foreign-looking moustache, beard or

RESPECT FOR ORNAMENTS IN TRADITIONAL styles, using objects found in the natural world, characterized the Hippies and lives on with the Modern Primitives. A wide range of 'ethnic' body decorations, especially from North American Indian, North African and Asian cultures, form the look. *left* Sharon wears ornaments from around the world and uses feathers, bone and amber; *opposite* henna artist Danny, with shell necklace and other, traditional 'ethnic'-style decorations

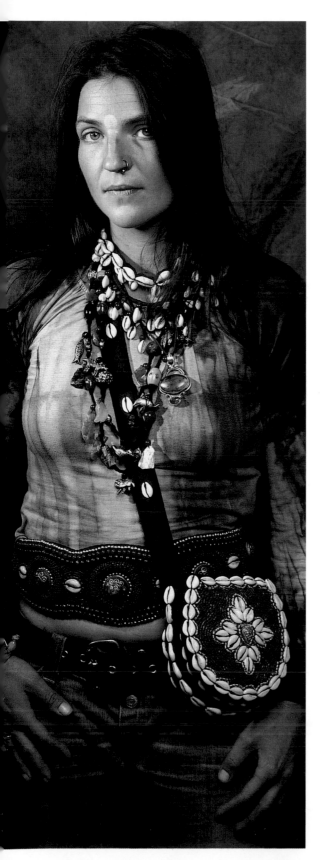

greased-back hairstyle. This is hardly surprising given the extremely limited scope available to Western men for any exuberance or creative leeway in transforming their physical appearance. Originally born of a fear that revolution might spread beyond France if the leisured aristocracy did not spin-doctor its image to resemble that of the hard-working, sober bourgeoisie, the ideal of the drab, visually unadventurous Invisible Man was further reinforced in the Age of Empire as a means of drawing a line between serious and 'civilized' Western men and, on the other hand, the often peacock-like natives they sought to subjugate. Thus Western man conquered the world, at the price of losing his own physicality. In time, as developing countries (as they would come to be called) sought to emulate the West, their own elite males discarded their traditional flamboyance and also embraced what the social historian J. C. Flugel termed 'The Great Masculine Renunciation' of sartorial finery and ostentatious body decoration. In the process, they cast aside a core component of their heritage; leaving them lost in a cultural no-man's-land between the West and their abandoned past.

Ironically (but, at least in retrospect, not surprisingly), the re-emergence of the peacock male took place not 'out there' but right at the urbane heart of Western civilization. The Bohemians of Paris, the Hipsters and Beats of New York, the Mods of Swinging London, the Rockabillies of Memphis, the Bikers and Hippies of San Francisco, all – in their own highly distinctive ways – sought to challenge the restricting legacy of the Invisible Man; to question the by then long-held view that a real man should be heard but not seen. All these subcultures had female as well as male members, but just as Western fashion has long been predominantly female territory, so such 'alternative' streetstyle has always had at its heart a celebration of male style.

While the scarcity of flamboyant adornment for Western men over the last two hundred years almost by definition labels any re-emergence of body decoration as exotic, it would be the Hippies, in the second half of the 1960s, who explicitly located the origins of their adornment styles outside the boundaries of Western civilization: prizing the fact that their embroidered headbands and fringing derived from North American Indian culture, their beads from Morocco, their bracelets and necklaces from India or Tibet.

By the end of the 1960s such exoticism would impact heavily on both high and mainstream fashion. At the same time, another product of the Hippies'

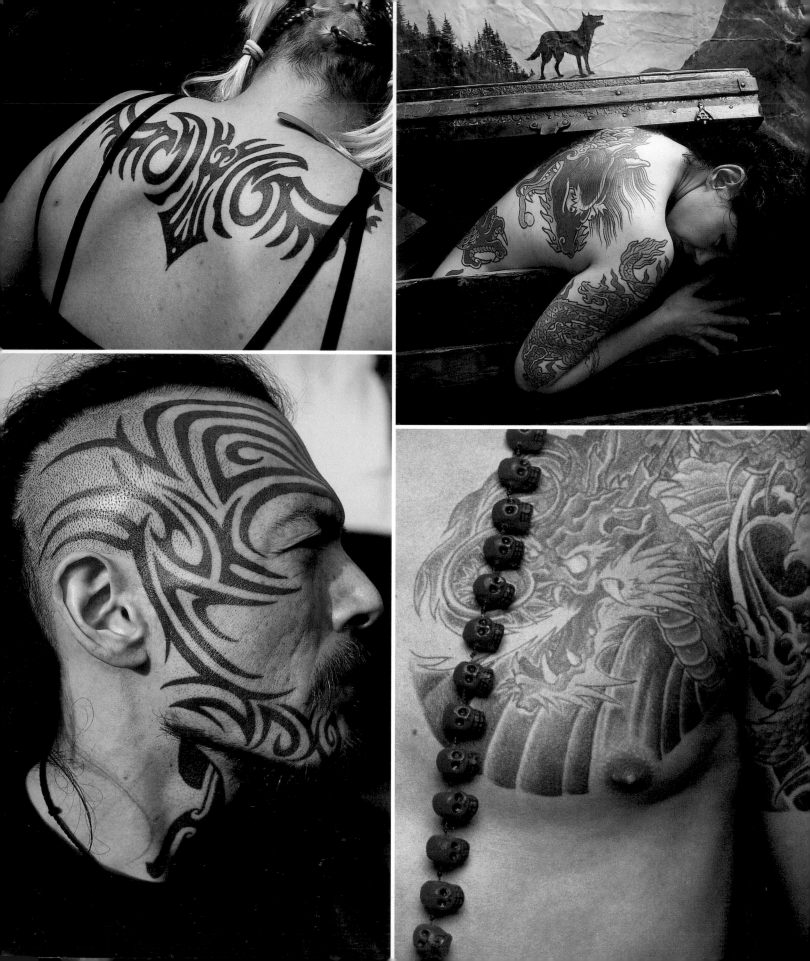

respect and fondness for all things ethnic and traditional (and one that seemed destined to retain its antifashion street credibility) came in the form of a renewed interest in the tattoo styles of the Pacific. As discussed in chapter two, while the West has its own ancient tattoo traditions, this particular form of permanent body decoration has long been seen in Europe and America as intrinsically exotic. The primarily West Coast-based pioneers of the tattoo renaissance took advantage of their geographic location to travel throughout the Pacific in order to learn more about the techniques and styles of tattooing practised in this part of the world. Back in America (and subsequently Europe, Australia and so on), especially within the receptive context of a typically middle-class, 'alternative' cultural environment, this knowledge of and enthusiasm for non-Western approaches to tattoo art became identified as Tribal and acquired a popularity that made it a cornerstone of the tattoo renaissance.

Starting in London in 1976, Punk explicitly paid homage to its tribal and primitive stylistic inspirations (in contrast to the Hippies, who had settled on a softer, ethnic aesthetic with peasant rather than primitive connotations). Unprecedented media attention – not to mention their own, often extremely provocative, on-the-street, in-your-face personal presence – brought the Punks' stylistic and ideological primitivism to everyone's attention. Europe's Surrealist and Cubist artists from the 1920s onwards had also found inspiration in primitive art, but in the Punks' case it was even more startling and (for many) disturbing because they applied such styles directly to that most intimate and provocative artistic medium, the human body.

While some Hippies copied North American Indian embroidery, fringing and headbands, the Punks (more radically) completely shaved some areas of their scalps, while using all manner of fixatives to create gravity-defying sections of hair, in a style that became known as Mohawk. Even more dramatically, they adopted a colour palette that contrasted graphic black with vibrant, fluorescent shades (for make-up and hair) reminiscent of those favoured by many of the natives of Amazonia (and some parts of Africa), which – while mimicking birds and reptiles – seem artificial in their brilliance. But the Punks' most breathtaking and controversial stylistic primitivism was their penchant for face and body piercing: for example, all around the rim of the ear, through the nostrils and septum of the nose, the cheeks and the lips. While most if not all of these piercings can be (or, probably more accurately, once were) found among

THE TATTOO RENAISSANCE

has brought new attention and respect to traditional tattoo styles from around the world but focused in particular on a wide range of styles from the Pacific. *opposite from top left, clockwise* Anne, with graphic Tribal back-piece; Marisa, with dragon tattoo in the Japanese style by Alex Binnie; Wesley, with Japanese chest tattoo based on a Yakuza design; Su'a Sulu'ape FreeWind, facial tattoo based primarily on Native North American Indian styles, blended with influences from Polynesia and Micronesia, by Leo Zulueta (one of the first great tattooists of the Neo Tribal style), and hand-tapped neck Tatau in Bornean style by Eddie David Kalum. A tattoo artist himself, he says: 'The term Tribal should be defined as having a direct visual, emotional and intuitive effect upon the viewer that would represent a feeling, story or ideology that suits its wearer and internal symbolism within the design that suggests a cultural origin as opposed to a polymorphic smashed tarantula that was unfortunately stuck on any part of the skin.'

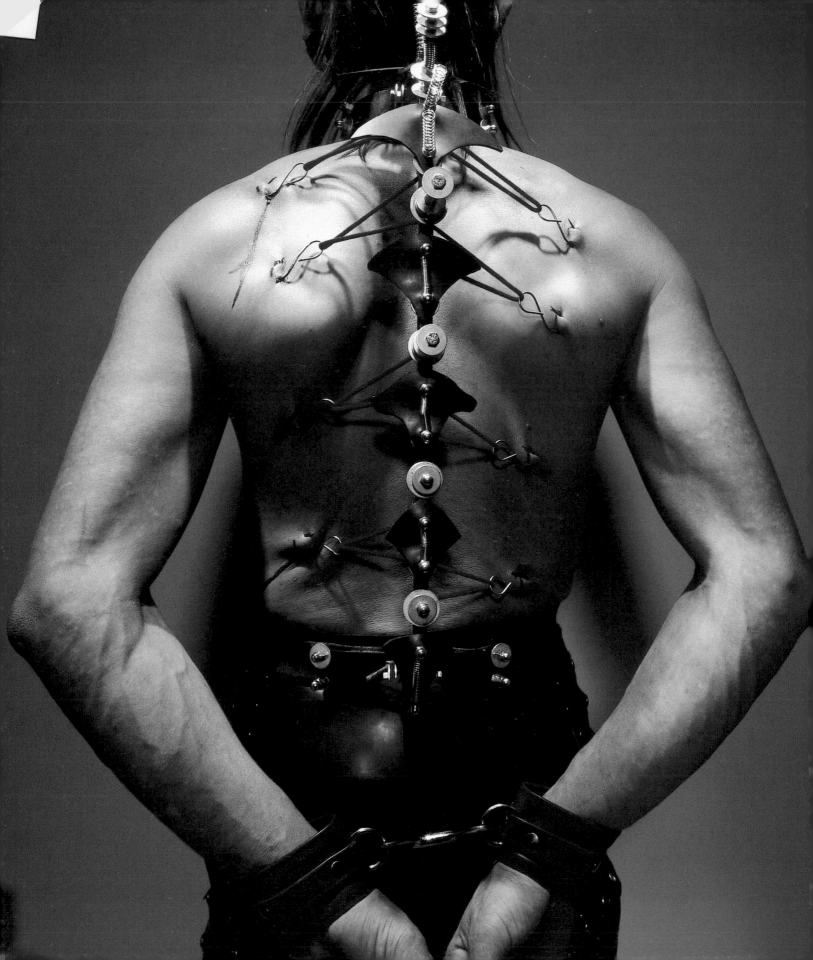

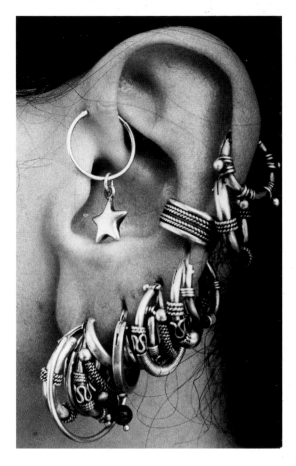

traditional peoples, the Punks' use of such things as humble safety pins gave them a personal style that demonstrated the principles of Postmodernism visually, long before many cultural theorists had grasped it conceptually.

Even more so than tattooing, piercing had all but disappeared from Western culture as a body art technique prior to this startling reintroduction by the Punks. Their piercings caught the attention of the media, but as discussed in chapter four, a small group of piercing enthusiasts was researching the ethnographic heritage of this body art in a more rigorous (and, from a health and safety point of view, more sound) fashion. Their work blossomed into a piercing renaissance that now includes thousands of full-time practitioners worldwide.

Another important body modification pioneer at this time, an American from South Dakota who settled in California and who chose to call himself Fakir Musafar (after a real-life 18th-century Persian 'Human Pincushion' featured in *Ripley's Believe It Or Not*), contributed a lifetime of detailed ethnographic research into scarification, tattooing and a host of other traditional techniques as well as piercing. Above and beyond his knowledge of ancient forms of body decoration, Musafar also brought a lifetime's fascination with how a great many traditional societies use painful techniques such as piercing in ritual, as a means of achieving altered states of consciousness. Identifying himself and those of similar inclinations as Modern Primitives, Musafar formalized and gave historical and ethnographic substance to the idea (first revered by the Hippies and the Punks) that there is benefit to be had from reaching back from a technologically advanced, but increasingly spiritually sterile, contemporary world to learn from traditional, exotic peoples. This often involves the enactment of traditional body rituals (for example the *O-Kee-Pa* ceremony of the Mandan and Sioux tribes during which a warrior would hang for hours from large hooks piercing his chest) to energize body, mind and spirit.

In 1989, the RE/Search book *Modern Primitives* introduced such thinking to a wider, international audience and there is a steadily growing tribe of people throughout the world who, as well as transforming their physical appearance using techniques and styles of body decoration that derive from primitive cultures, are experimenting with extreme, painful (and, to an outsider's eye, often disturbing) rituals of body modification. (These modifications are sometimes only intended as temporary, as it is often the ritual experience itself rather than the permanent decoration of the body that is sought.)

THE ACT OF ACQUIRING A PIERCING,
the ritual process, is for many at least as important as the decorative result. Modern Primitives in particular are looking back to ancient North American Indian culture for inspiration for deliberately painful but, it is thought, consciousness-raising and spiritually enhancing body rituals. *opposite* Marcel, piercing performance back corset with metal spine; *above* more is more – multiple ear piercings

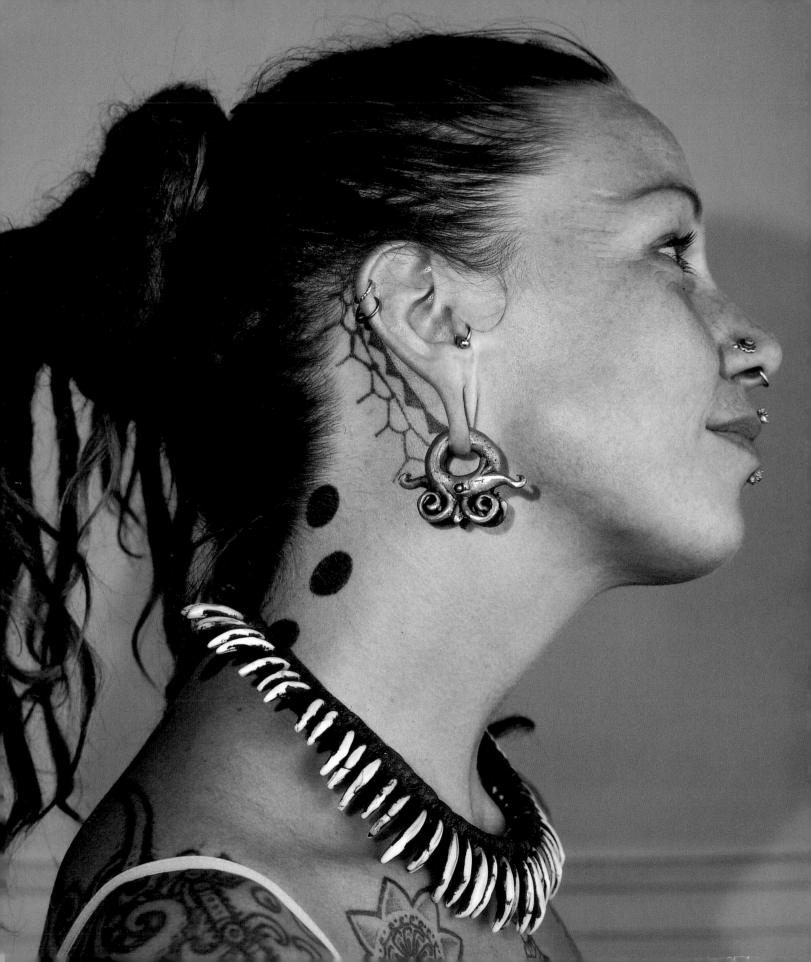

Although the number of those who would explicitly identify themselves as Modern Primitives is large it remains a minority subculture. However, albeit in a less extreme (and unarticulated) form, this yearning after the primitive – the most extreme of all exotic tendencies; seeking out those ways of life most distant – pervades Western culture today. In the sphere of body decoration (the most visible application of this world view) it clearly plays a significant part in the phenomenal rise in popularity of piercing and tattooing (though its influence can also be found in face and body painting, hairstyling, the increased popularity of henna decoration and styles of non-piercing ornament). Increasingly, the decorated body is not only exotic in character, but specifically tribal and primitive in its styling and associations. The ultimate in exoticism, the Modern Primitive inclination not only takes people all the way 'out there' but, also, as far as it is possible to travel in the imagination, 'back there' to the very origins of our species.

The (Post) Modern Primitive is a logical impossibility. The ever greater complexity and ever quicker pace of change in today's world create an impossible environment for any true application of traditional values. The idea that acquiring a Tribal piercing, tattoo or hairstyle can catapult us into some Amazonian or Polynesian idyll is clearly absurd. Yet it must also be said that, in the midst of the alienation, anomie and inauthenticity that is the Postmodern condition, we would be well advised to learn whatever we can from those cultures that perfected socially stabilizing and, apparently, spiritually satisfying ways of being. We know from anthropological studies that the vast majority of such primitive peoples found painful rite of passage rituals and permanent body decorations of sufficient value that they saw fit to institutionalize and hold on to these practices throughout their long histories. Rather than a sporadic occurrence, permanent, painful transformations of appearance such as tattooing, scarification and piercing were in fact a consistent feature of most tribal societies – as early explorers and anthropologists noted and that scores of missionaries fought against. It was in this way that the social body (the tribal group) and personal, individual experience interacted to create what so persistently eludes us today – a meaningful matrix of reality.

Thus, with the spread of Postmodern Primitivism, the world reaches a curious juncture at which Westerners respect and covet as never before those same body decorations that most of the traditional cultures that first created

TODAY'S MODERN PRIMITIVE,
unlike a member of a traditional society, can sample and mix different adornment styles from cultures worldwide and throughout history. Ironically, therefore, neither modern nor primitive, this group exemplifies a Postmodern eclecticism that is neither here nor there, now nor then. *opposite* Modern Primitive Vicky, Belgium, with scarification at the sides of her eyes, stretched and other ear piercings, nose and lip piercings, dreads, tattoos and necklace made from natural materials

them seem set on dispensing with in the pursuit of modernity (which, to complete the circular irony, the West is already 'post'). An earlier model of this bizarre situation occurred in Japan just after it was forcibly obliged to open itself to the West: while humble sailors and European aristocrats alike flocked there to acquire tattoos at the hands of the country's great masters of the art, its own citizens were prohibited from being tattooed for fear that Japan would appear unsophisticated to Western eyes. Today, while some Third World governments have taken steps to discourage their citizens from acquiring traditional body decorations (as has happened with tribal scarification in parts of Africa), the more typical scenario is that of younger generations increasingly disinclined to submit to the permanent body modification rituals of their parents and ancestors. Their motivation is to be modern, progressive, urbane and Western.

Imagine, however, the shock and cultural confusion that must occur when, for example, a European, American or Australian tourist shows up in, say, Borneo wishing to be tattooed in the native, traditional style (or, indeed, wants to learn how to execute such designs on his or her customers back home). Perhaps, after an initial response of pure and utter amazement, such increasingly common occurrences will eventually promote a more positive reassessment by young, would-be Westernized generations of their own cultural heritage. Beyond this (as has apparently already happened in some places in the Pacific) such flattering emulation may also come to be seen as a form of cultural theft.

This is a serious issue. Designs and styles of body decoration constitute a key focal point for traditional cultures. In many instances, robbed of their native land and/or its natural wealth, decimated by disease and flight to urban centres, such ancient cultures have little else to bind them together and to their proud past. Thus, in the eyes of some traditional peoples, today's Modern Primitive or exotically decorated tourist is simply a new form of imperialist. In a sense they are right. Decorations in many cases were traditionally worn only by adult members of a particular tribe (and, often, only those whose leadership or bravery in battle or hunting had earned them the right). Furthermore, for a Westerner to choose a traditional tattoo, scarification or other form of body modification simply because it looks nice is to take something of great symbolic resonance and demote it to the status of a nearly meaningless decoration.

CAN THE ESSENTIAL CONSERVATISM and cultural specificity of traditional societies coexist with today's increasingly fast-changing and global way of life? Responding to the perceived spiritual poverty and cultural confusion of contemporary life, the Modern Primitive movement attempts to learn from and – literally in its body decorations – incorporate the values of traditional cultures. *opposite* Modern Primitive Chico, Bulgaria, with North American Indian and other adornments including feathers and bone

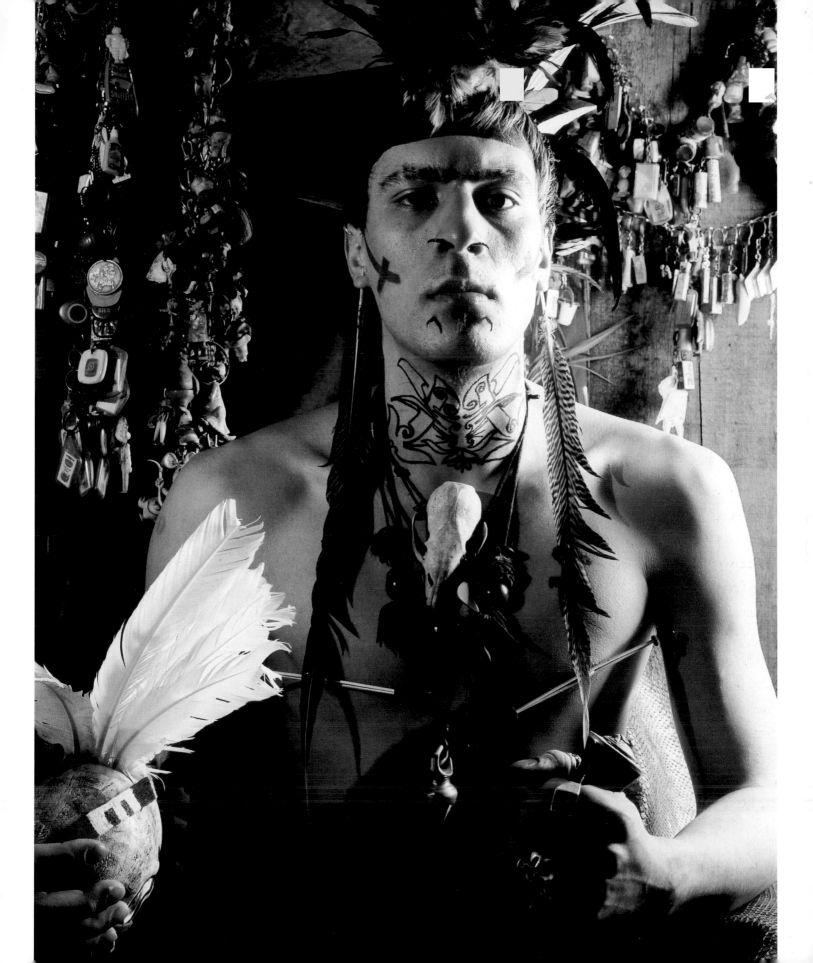

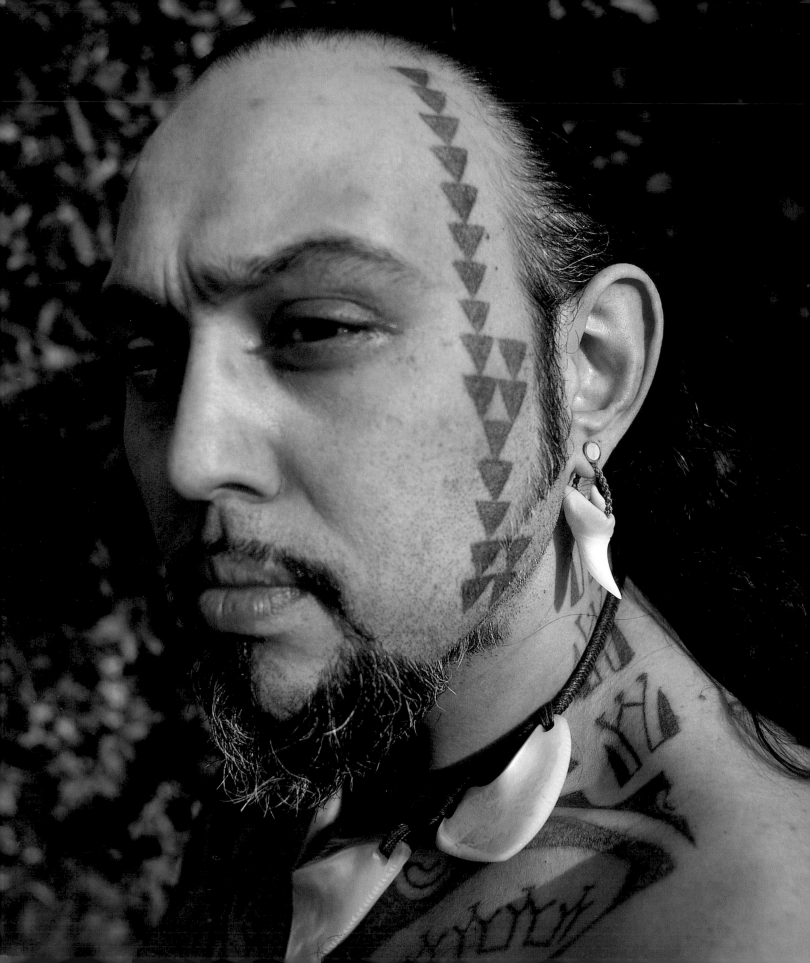

THE CURRENT POPULARITY OF TRIBAL
body decoration is the most visible evidence of a
shift in Western worldview from arrogance to respect.
But should traditional societies charge Westerners
a copyright fee? *opposite* Tangaroatuane, New Zealand,
Hawaiian facial tattoo by Kione Nunes, who learned from
Paolo Su'a Sulu'ape: 'To my ancestors, the preservation
of life through genealogy, the art of *moko*, was more
valuable than all the riches of the world'; *below* Tribal
influence in tattoos, with Western dress, Amsterdam

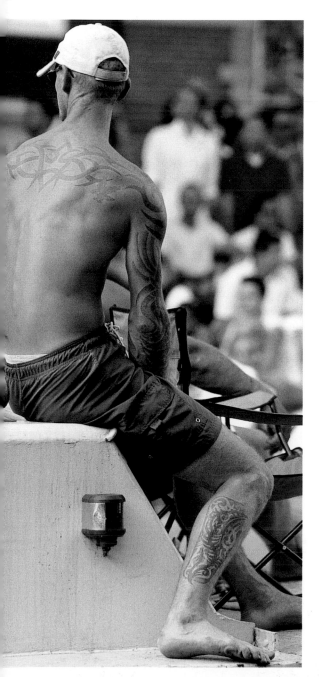

On the other hand, however, after centuries of Western arrogance and presumption that the West alone possesses culture and civilization, is not that humble respect that undoubtedly lies at the heart of the current interest in the exotic and primitive to be valued and welcomed? There may be some for whom the attraction is purely aesthetic and only skin deep, but for many more it is deeper, philosophical – reflecting an awareness that, far from possessing a monopoly on wisdom, Western culture's inadequacies are all too clearly apparent.

This is a useful message to send to those younger members of traditional societies who, in the glare and glitz of global culture, may see only the positive and miss the negative realities of 'progress'. And, on the other side of the fence, at a time when the West so evidently doesn't know where it is headed (the Modernist locomotive derailed but still hurtling forward), is it not valuable and responsible to consider other, older lifestyle options? Contemporary global culture is but one experiment in living – and, indeed, one still in its infancy and untested by time. Traditional, primitive cultures began conducting their own, separate experiments long ago and collectively discovered in body ritual and decoration an invaluable tool for the construction of meaning and reality. In its highly unusual (not to say downright perverse) bifurcation of mind and body, the Western world view made it extremely difficult to see that we are intrinsically holistic beings – to value physicality and, therefore, the human body as a medium of artistic expression. Perhaps, then, the passionate, heady embrace of The Exotic Body – and now especially its ultimate form, The Primitive Body – is simply the only means left to us to climb back into our own skins.

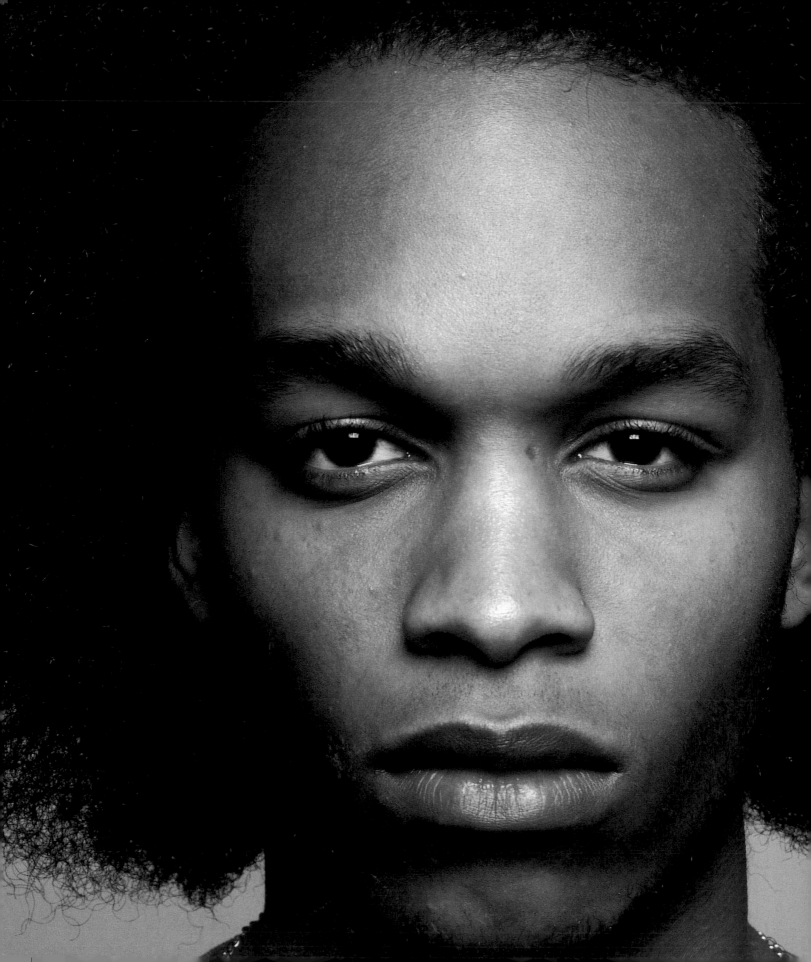

CHAPTER SEVEN
THE ARTIFICIAL BODY

A great many of the things human beings do to transform their appearance are not body decoration per se because they are performed in the hope that such transformations will be invisible to others. As well as plastic surgery, a principal if not majority component of the global beauty industry falls within this category of non-decorative transformations of appearance, for example: natural-look skin creams, foundations, blushers, tanning lotions, nail polish, lipgloss and hair dyes. For many women (and a steadily rising percentage of men) it is normal practice to spend substantial amounts of time and money in order to look as if you'd not spent a second or a penny on your appearance. Indeed, the Natural Look (in which the body is presented as if untouched by man-made products or techniques) is arguably the most popular style option available today.

As even a cursory review of beauty (in traditional societies or throughout most of Western history) clearly demonstrates, a naturalistic ideal is the exception rather than the rule for our species. Body painting, tattooing, scarification, piercing, ornamentation, hairstyling and so forth have the common goal of explicitly making visible and celebrating the artificial manipulation – the artistry – that has been applied to the body. To expend great effort and cost (and, as in many forms of plastic surgery, to endure considerable pain) to achieve an appearance that – if successful – erases all trace of that effort, cost and pain, would seem very strange to a traditional society in which the point of transforming the

ARGUABLY THE MOST POPULAR
body style – a naturalistic ideal.
this page Martin, with Natural Look Afro

body is the visible decoration (the scarification, the teeth filed into sharp points, the razored scalp) that results from the transforming process.

Perhaps some members of Western society so vigorously pursue an ideal of natural beauty for the simple reason that, for the first time in human history, the level of technological sophistication is such that they can. Never before has it been possible to produce such effective antiwrinkle creams, foundations that conceal defects while blending into the skin, or hair dyes that so perfectly mimic shades found in nature that as in the popular advertisements of the 1960s 'Only Your Hairdresser Knows For Sure'. Even more astounding are the advances that have been made in plastic surgery – advances that now make it possible to transform the shape and appearance of the human body in ways traditional peoples (not to mention our great-grandparents) would have found completely unbelievable.

To focus exclusively on our technological sophistication in these matters would be to miss an important point. In their own way, traditional peoples devised what were – in their time and place – mind-boggling techniques for transforming physical appearance: stretching piercings to accommodate enormous plugs, laying designs of tattoos or raised scars over large areas of flesh, dramatically altering the shape of infants' skulls or, famously, as among the Padaung people of Burma, stretching the length of the neck. In none of these, however, or all the other countless instances that might be cited, was the objective a naturalistic beauty ideal. To be sure, such transformations were always seen as making the individual more attractive, but (and this is the important point) this beauty was always explicitly valued as artificial – a product of culture rather than birth. For ironically, while we tend to see traditional (especially tribal) peoples as more natural than ourselves ('Natural Savages' as previous generations put it) they themselves rejoiced in their artifice; the degree of distance from nature they achieved seen as the marker of their cultural accomplishment and civilization. And nowhere was this more evident (or purposeful) than in their body decoration.

Against this backdrop, Western culture's fascination with the natural emerges as distinctive, even peculiar. And far from being a minority or only contemporary concern, this yearning for unsullied nature is to be found right at the heart of Judeo-Christian culture: seeing humankind's departure from the pure naturalism of the Garden of Eden as tragic estrangement rather than

ARTIFICE IN APPEARANCE is natural to our species – and modification universal. No society has ever been found in which it is the norm simply to let nature run its course in determining appearance. Unlike other animals, human beings have always sought to transform and decorate themselves, often in startling ways. *opposite* Martin, who appears on the previous pages with a Natural Look Afro, is here transformed with make-up and floral head-piece

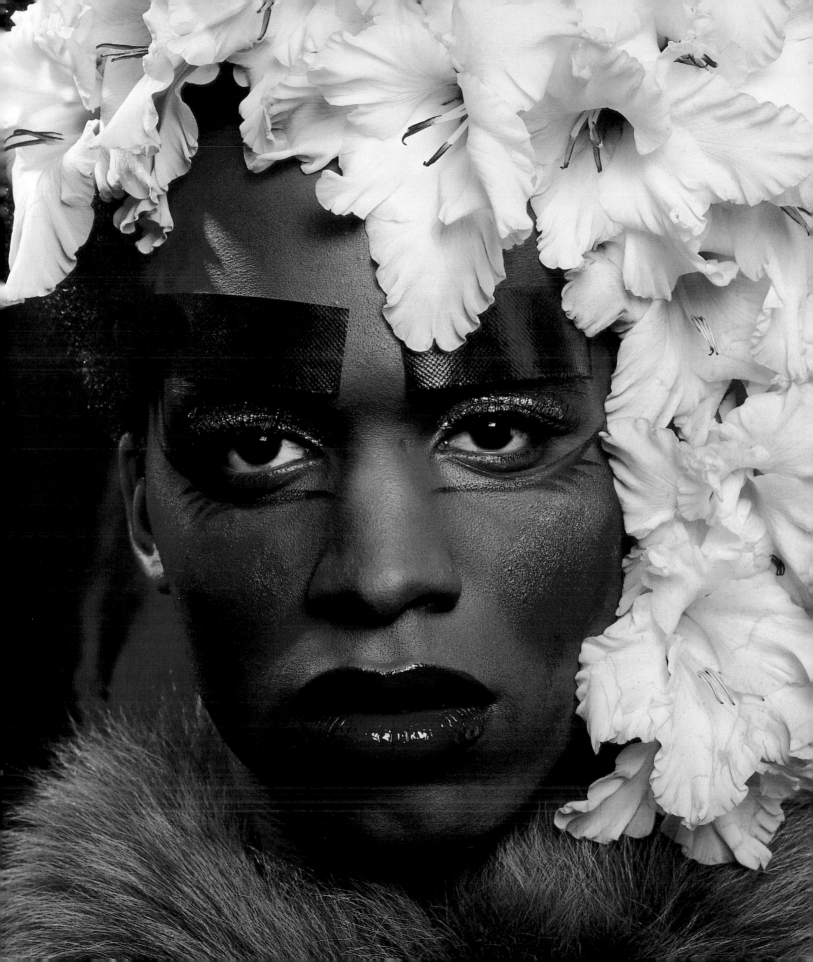

proud achievement. Rousseau's love affair with 'The Noble Savage' picked up on this theme, and while Europe sent countless missionaries to convert the heathen, its envy of these peoples' apparent naturalness couldn't be concealed. The Industrial Revolution's pollution and environmental damage offered tangible proof not only of man's distance from nature but also his capacity to destroy it. Reacting against this, industrial progress was matched by a romanticizing of the countryside and a pronounced shift towards a more naturalistic personal appearance style for both men and women.

In the 20th century the creed of naturalism found its ultimate, most widespread realization when it became the cornerstone of the Hippies' world view and found expression in a style positioned as far as possible from the artificial looks (white lipstick, thick, jet-black mascara, bright plastic jewelry, lacquered, teased, towering or sharp-edged geometric hairstyles, fun fashion wigs) that had been so popular in the first half of the 1960s. For a time in 1966 or 1967, things were poised in a nearly equal balance between futuristic artifice (the high fashion influence of Paco Rabanne, Pierre Cardin, Betsey Johnson or Rudi Gernreich's sci-fi experiments; *Barbarella*; Pop Art; James Bond movie sets and gadgets) and the earthy, casual naturalistic look that the Hippies saw as 'real' as opposed to 'plastic' (the ultimate Hippy term of abuse). By the end of the 1960s the Hippies' naturalism had tipped the balance to become the more powerful force. Artifice became increasingly suspect – especially for women, for whom make-up and fancy hairstyles were increasingly viewed as anti-feminist as well as plastic. Thus, interestingly, whereas the first half of the 1960s had experienced unisex in the form of more men experimenting with feminine adornments, now, in the second half, unisex more typically resulted from women becoming more masculine – giving up noticeable decoration and adornment. Within a short period of time the Natural Look broke free of its street origins to impact on both high fashion and mainstream beauty ideals where, to this day, it exerts great influence – Natural recognized as a perennially popular style option.

Within this exaltation of the natural it is often difficult to keep in mind that the idea of natural beauty is itself a cultural construction. In a different time, in a different society (or even subculture), distinct, often contradictory definitions of natural beauty will be found. Unlike other animals, we are not born with a defined standard, an instinctive template of physical perfection: we acquire,

THE NATURAL LOOK,
unique to the West and to recent times, in truth
may be achieved using the latest, most advanced
cosmetic technology. Going further, the ultimate
tool in the search for 'natural beauty', extraordinary
advances in plastic surgery now make it possible to
alter permanently almost every feature of appearance.
Yet ideals of beauty are always a product of culture and
history. *right* Charelene provides one interpretation
of the Natural Look

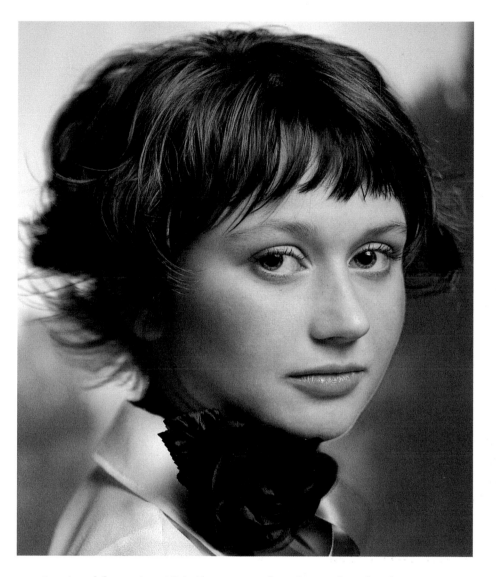

construct and deconstruct it in the course of our lives. What the plastic surgeon
offers as the must-have, most naturally beautiful shape for nose, lips, breasts or
bottom today may have to be undone or reversed at a later date. Furthermore,
in an increasingly heterogeneous society (or, more precisely, the cheek by jowl
clustering of lots of different societies), your definition of beauty may be your
neighbour's definition of ugliness. And let us not forget the profound irony of
the fact that the pursuit of natural beauty increasingly involves astounding
technological and scientific achievement.

Natural is a look, a style rather than a biological bottom line. And, like all
appearance styles, it visualizes and encodes a particular, utopian world view –
a politics – of how human life might, ideally, be lived. The Hippies' particular
vision of the Garden of Eden – The Age of Aquarius – accommodated some

HOWEVER FUTURISTIC ARTIFICIAL STYLES
may appear, they are also inevitably reminiscent of
the extraordinary appearance styles created long
ago by tribal peoples. *overleaf* D-Monica and Chico
wear ultraviolet face and hair paint for a techno party

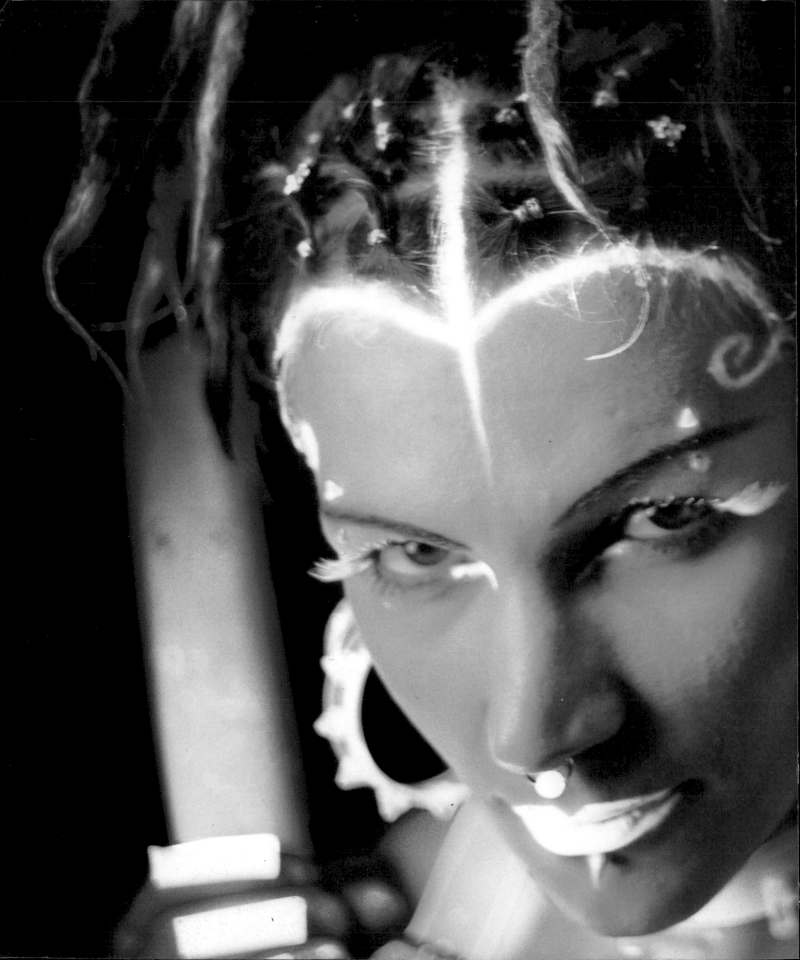

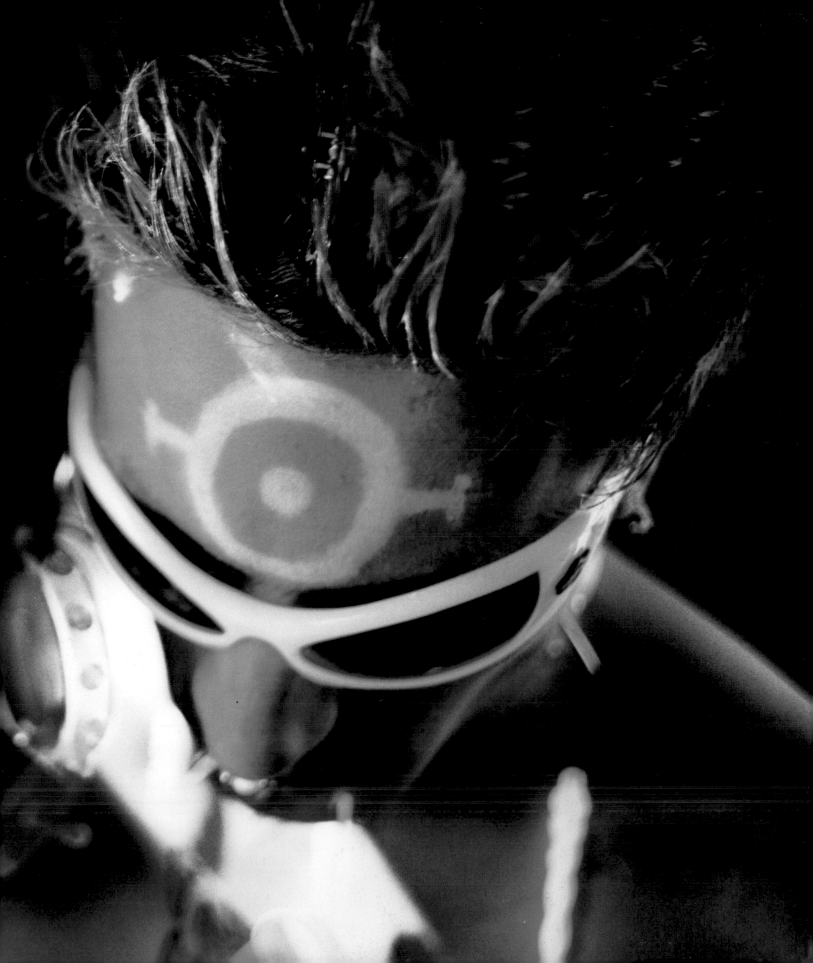

ethnic (non-Western) decorations (Moroccan beads, North American Indian headbands, henna hair dyes) as suitably natural while finding other ethnographic sources of inspiration (for example many of the tribal peoples of the Amazon, Africa and the Pacific) unacceptable because the vivid, fluorescent colour palette favoured by many of these peoples (which the Punks would delight in) seemed too pop, plastic and unreal. Natural is always a fiction because the only thing that is truly natural for human beings is artifice. (And let us not forget that 'natural beauty' is a tool that helps ruling elites to maintain their superiority over other classes, races, ethnic and religious groups.)

Today, the Natural Look is but one of many style options that coexist within our age's Postmodern supermarket of style. Despite a brief flirtation with naturalism, most of fashion quickly rediscovered its long-standing love affair – indeed, its marriage of convenience – with artifice. In terms of streetstyle, while the Mods' and Psychedelics' delight in artifice was eclipsed by late 1960s naturalistic fervour, it reasserted itself with a vengeance with the advent of Glam in the early 1970s. From the extraterrestrial presence of Ziggy Stardust and his vivid, always decidedly unnatural colleagues, a lineage can be traced through the Punks, the New Romantics, the Goths and – via Rave and Techno – right up to the brightly painted, glittering bodies of participants in Berlin's most recent Love Parade.

Artifice too is a style, a look, an aesthetic option. Like the natural, it is a signification that points beyond itself to suggest a vision, a philosophy of how life ideally might be. In the early 1960s, artificial style existed as a shorthand for the delights of a future age when technological advances would free humankind from drudgery and illness, while liberation from dated and unnecessary inhibitions and social mores would free the spirit for previously unimagined delights. Like the streetstyles of the Mods and Psychedelics, Glam also equated artifice with futurism – raising the prospect of gender, as well as sexual, freedom – but, in its most prescient moments, giving a foretaste of Postmodernism's wariness about what the future might hold.

Of course the Punks delighted in artifice – if for no other reason than that it offered the perfect counterpoint to the leftover naturalism of the leftover Hippies of the mid-1970s. But, at the same time, their core value of (now thoroughly Postmodern) cynicism and irony required them to also ditch wide-eyed enthusiasm for progress and the presumption that things could only

NEW TECHNOLOGY TODAY

has created techniques for transforming appearance that have never before been dreamt possible, despite truly mind-boggling techniques such as the huge lip plates of the Amazon, scarification in Africa, tattooing in the Pacific, sharply pointed skulls in Mesoamerica and stretched necks in Southeast Asia. *opposite from top left, clockwise* Iris wearing black contact lenses; Marcel transforms himself into an alien being with the aid of jewelry, make-up and piercings; Ursula, with modified 'Captain Spock' ear; D-Monica, with techno party face decorations and jewelry

THE POSTMODERN AGE

embraces extremes of both naturalism and artifice. Never before have such divergent ideals of beauty and desire coexisted at the same time. In both cases extraordinary technologies are brought to bear to achieve the desired result. But while plastic surgery and other Natural Look techniques strive to remain invisible, cutting-edge experimentors in artifice such as Silver AJ, *overleaf*, proudly display the technology of their appearance style

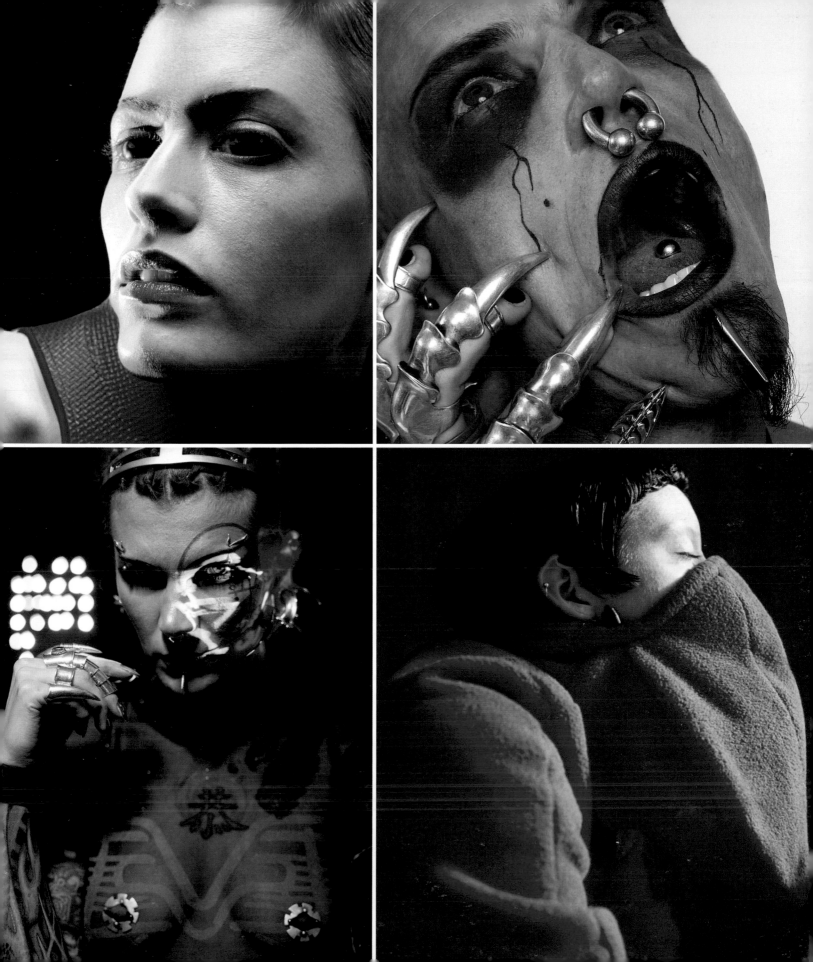

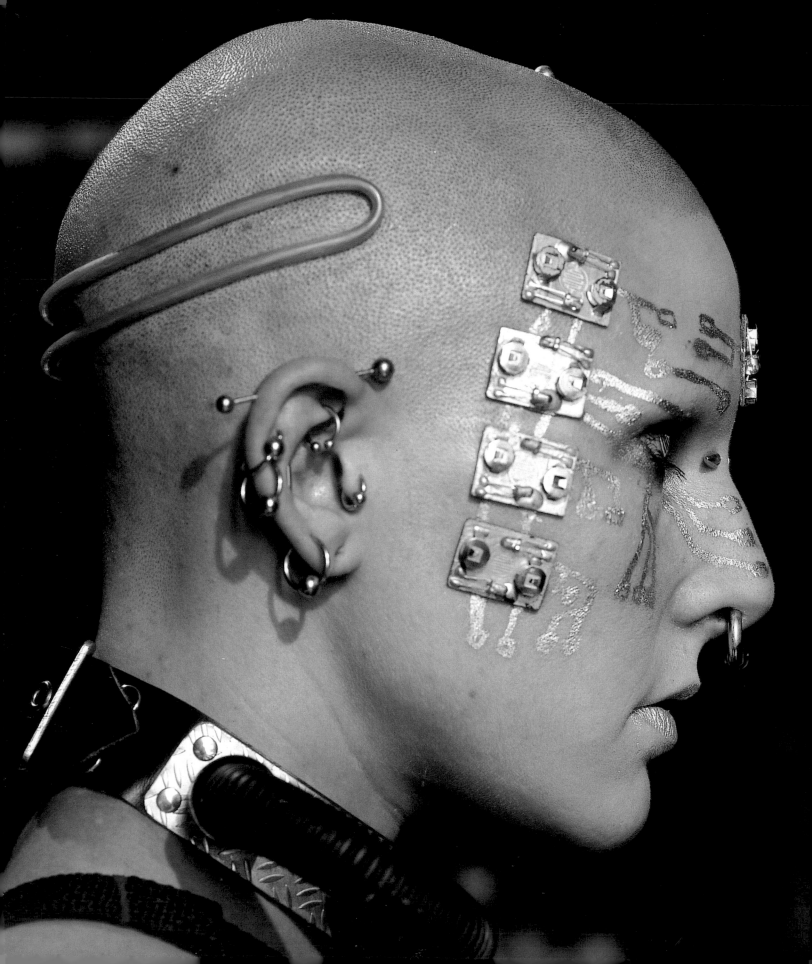

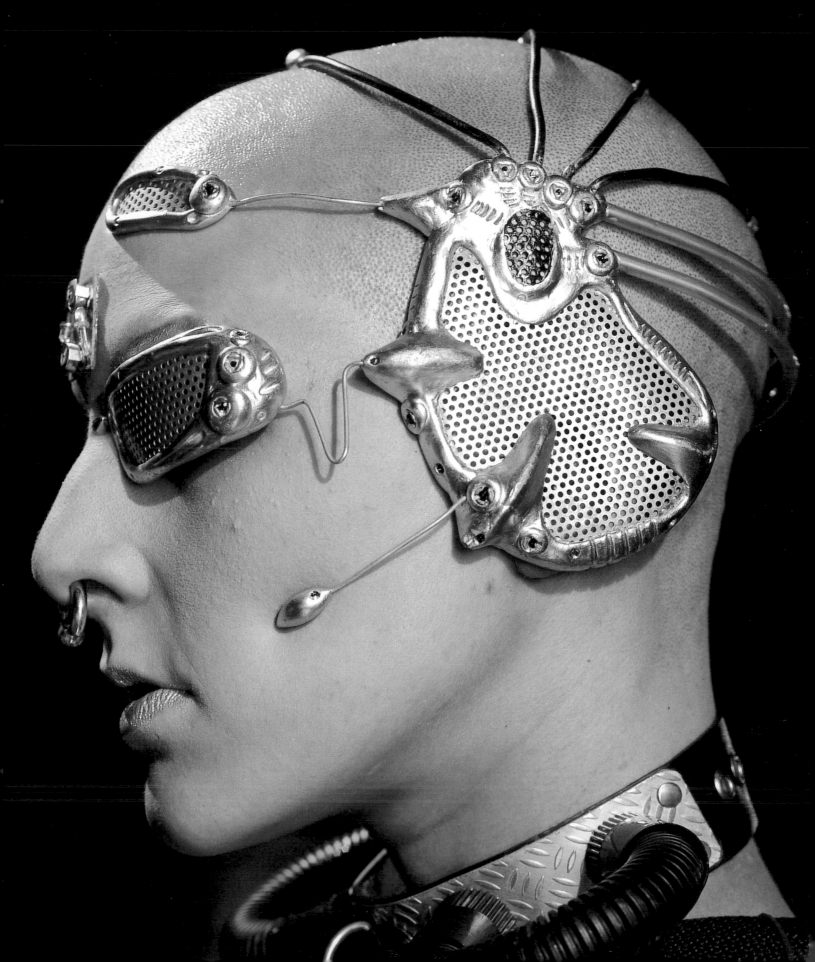

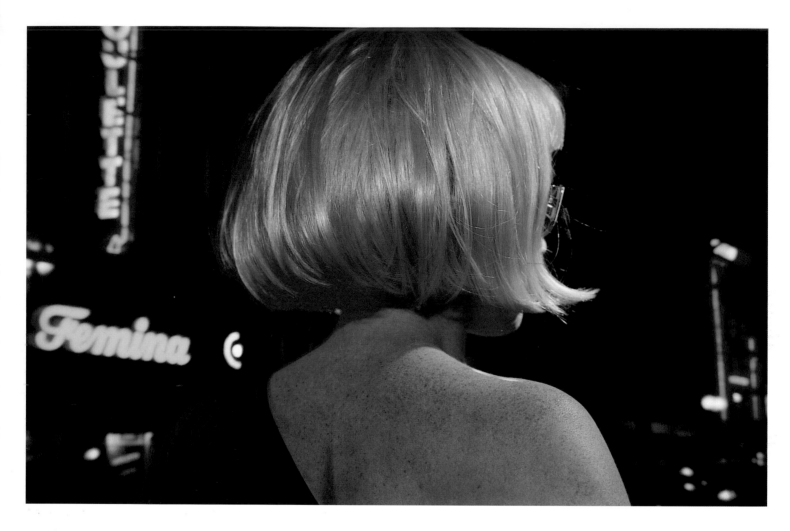

get better. This 'No Future' futurism re-encoded artifice into a trashy kitsch look/attitude that took perverse delight in the sexy dystopia Ziggy Stardust and the Spiders from Mars had first glimpsed on the horizon.

Punk also – uniquely at the time – grasped that extreme eclecticism that would become the other defining feature of the Postmodern condition. Accordingly, they brought to the party a whole array of different takes on artifice: as well as futurism and kitsch, a rediscovery of primitive unnaturalness. In this (the one and only point on which the Punks permitted themselves to put aside their cynicism) they stepped back in time to explore and embrace (with respect) a vision of human origins not all that far from Rousseau's 'Noble Savage'. In their Mohican hair, their piercings, their tattoos and their graphic make-up designs they saw what Arnold Rubin would later term *Marks of Civilization* – traces of meaningfulness that, like hardy bacteria clinging to life in a seemingly inhospitable environment, might survive even within the unreality

WE CHOOSE HOW TO PRESENT OURSELVES
to the world, often happily switching between one look and another – even Natural and artificial – for different occasions or different moods. *above* Joleen: 'This is my trashy blonde Dolly wig for incognito good times.'

and senselessness of the Postmodern age. As discussed in the previous chapter, this attitude of the Punks can be recognized in the Modern Primitive movement, which has impacted on both fashion and mainstream style to make even permanent Tribal body decorations a normal feature of life today. Interestingly, as with the Hippies' acceptance of body decorations and ornament that had a sufficiently ethnic pedigree, many people who see fashionable or glamorous styles of body decoration as unacceptable because of their presumed artificiality (and/or anti-feminist message) feel free to cover their bodies with tattoos or piercings, which they exempt from classification as artificial by virtue of their ancient and non-Western origins.

While only a few decades ago Western culture was characterized by dramatic pendulum swings back and forth between the natural and the artificial (Romanticism/Fin de Siècle decadence; the Hippies/Glam Rock), it is now characterized by the simultaneous embrace of both of these styles/philosophies, which exist simply as separate entrées on the Postmodern menu. Popstar/fashion designer/actor A opts for the Natural Look while popstar/fashion designer/actor B exalts artifice. Indeed, today a single individual can move even from one day to the next between these once seemingly antipodal positions without apparent psychic contradiction. Cultural theorists warn that the Postmodern age has lost all possibility of meaning, that we can no longer know when we have left the boundaries of the themepark. Beyond doubt, this jump-cutting nonchalantly between even nature and artifice – arguably, Western history's greatest discourse, for it incorporates the problematic dualities of nature/nurture and mind/body – offers incontrovertible proof that they are right. Yet, at the same time, to appreciate that nature and artifice are simply two sides of the same coin, alternative style options, is to come of age, to grasp what our ancestors knew long ago: reality is a matrix of our own construction. Far from being alarmingly schizophrenic, it is a reassuring cultural breakthrough – the moment when we wake up to the fact that everything we behold is an illusion, a construction. That this is even true of our own bodies, their perceived beauty or ugliness, their desires, pleasures and pains, is the final – most difficult but also most liberating – step in this discovery.

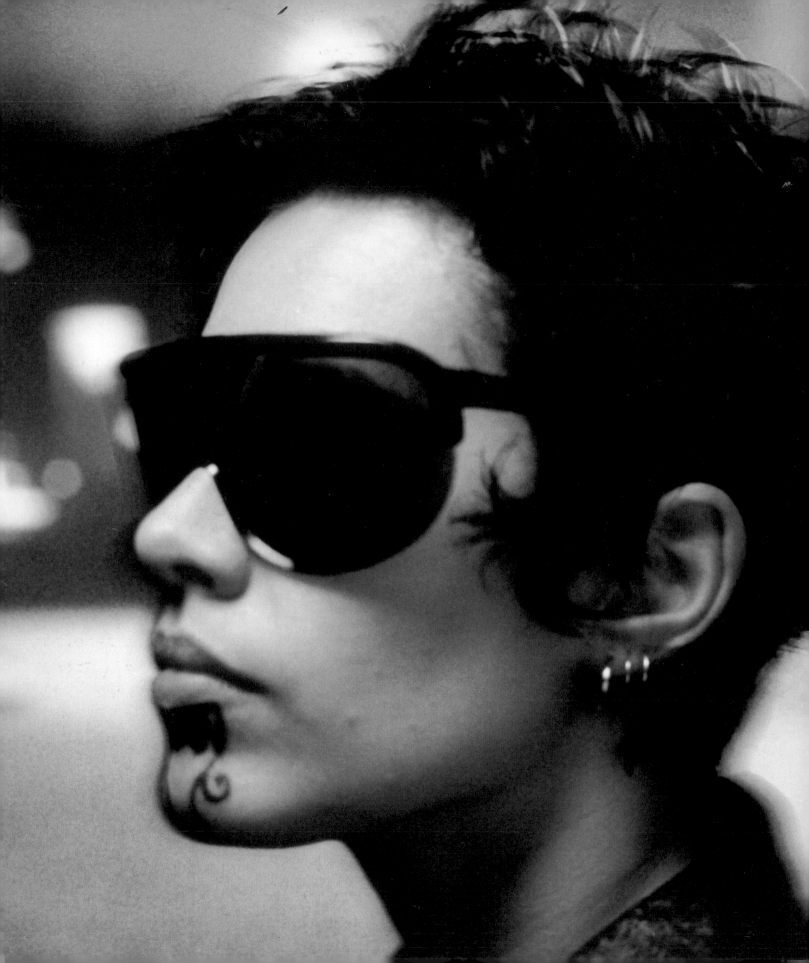

CHAPTER EIGHT

THE DO-IT-YOURSELF BODY

Beyond doubt, ours is the most exciting era in the entire, long history of body decoration. Nothing so extraordinary has happened since that seminal moment at least seventy thousand years ago when some distant ancestor discovered that his or her appearance could be transformed with markings of black soot or vivid red ochre. What makes the tail end of the 20th and start of the 21st centuries so distinctive is this: never before have there been so many techniques and styles from which to choose and – crucially – never before have we had such freedom in making these choices. Amazingly, this has all happened in the equivalent of a nanosecond of human history – a few decades.

When, beginning in the 1960s, a group of American tattooists began experimenting with new or newly rediscovered approaches to tattoo art, this was heralded as the tattoo renaissance. But the idea of a rebirth is now applicable to an ever-wider range of techniques for transforming appearance. In addition to tattooing we must include the astonishing explosion of interest in body piercing, a broader, more creative understanding of jewelry, the phenomenal development of the miniature masterpieces of nail art, radical experiments in tooth adornment and the apparently limitless new (or, again, newly rediscovered) possibilities for hairstyling and make-up.

The result of all these simultaneous innovations in the art of body decoration – and what truly sets our era apart – is the unprecedented freedom to remake ourselves into whatever

COMBINING ANCIENT AND FUTURISTIC in the DIY body. *these pages* Laurian, *moko*-style chin tattoo with sunglasses image we like. Throughout most of human history, traditional culture set strict, incontestable guidelines for acceptable appearance styles. A Maori chief could use only particular designs in his facial tattoo; a Sioux warrior could use only certain feathers in his headdress; all of the adult women of a New Guinea tribe would paint their bodies in exactly the same colours.

When the adornments of all traditional peoples are viewed collectively, we see a breathtaking range of styles and techniques for reinventing the human body. But we mustn't forget that such a cross-cultural overview is only possible from the privileged, international perspective of global culture. Within a particular traditional culture (and therefore throughout most of human history) the freedom to experiment with new forms, techniques and styles of adornment was rarely enjoyed. Intensely conservative and conformist, body decoration in such societies was regulated by and functioned for the sake of the group rather than, as in the contemporary era, the individual.

In Europe, from the 15th century onwards, it was fashion that introduced a radically different approach to appearance – one that changed systematically and quickly over time. But, in laying down strict guidelines on what was 'in' and what was 'out', fashion also severely restricted the possibilities for personal expression in appearance. A few decades ago, however, when first a minority and then a majority – eager to use dress and body decoration to make a personal statement rather than, as previously, to conform to one accepted new look – revolted against the totalitarian dictatorship of fashion, the result was a dramatic withering away of the rules governing appearance. Thus, even if some beauty editors persist in announcing with as much fanfare as they can muster what colour of lipstick or eyeshadow is 'in', few now pay much attention, and cosmetic manufacturers know that to succeed today they must produce an ever-expanding palette of colours and shades to cater to individual tastes. The same approach – in which the consumer's own creative choice prevails – now applies to hairstyling, nail art, jewelry and any of the other aspects of body decoration that previously were simply swept along in the tide of fashion.

Today we find ourselves within a kaleidoscopic supermarket of style where the options are apparently unlimited. Sampling and mixing colours and decorative techniques from different historical eras, geographic areas, other cultures and our own subcultures, we increasingly create our own distinctive, personal style statement rather than presenting ourselves as sheep-like

THE INDIVIDUAL CONSTRUCTS A UNIQUE appearance style that announces his or her personal identity, philosophy and dreams, escaping the anonymity of homogenized culture, and no longer subject to fashion dictates. *opposite* Rui

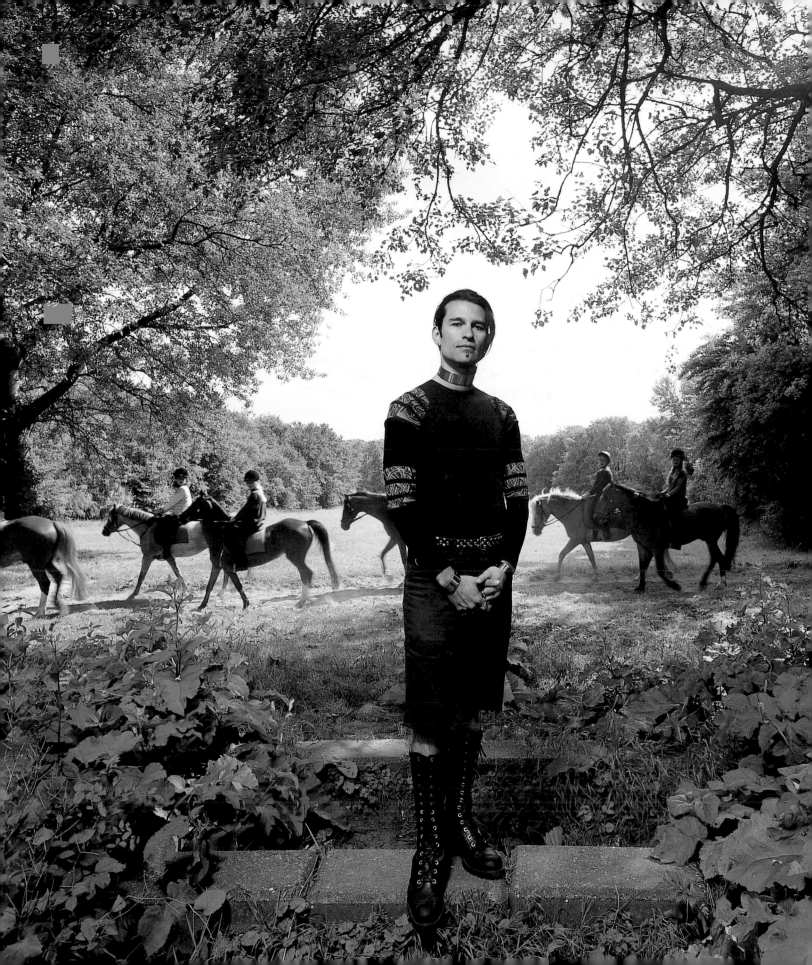

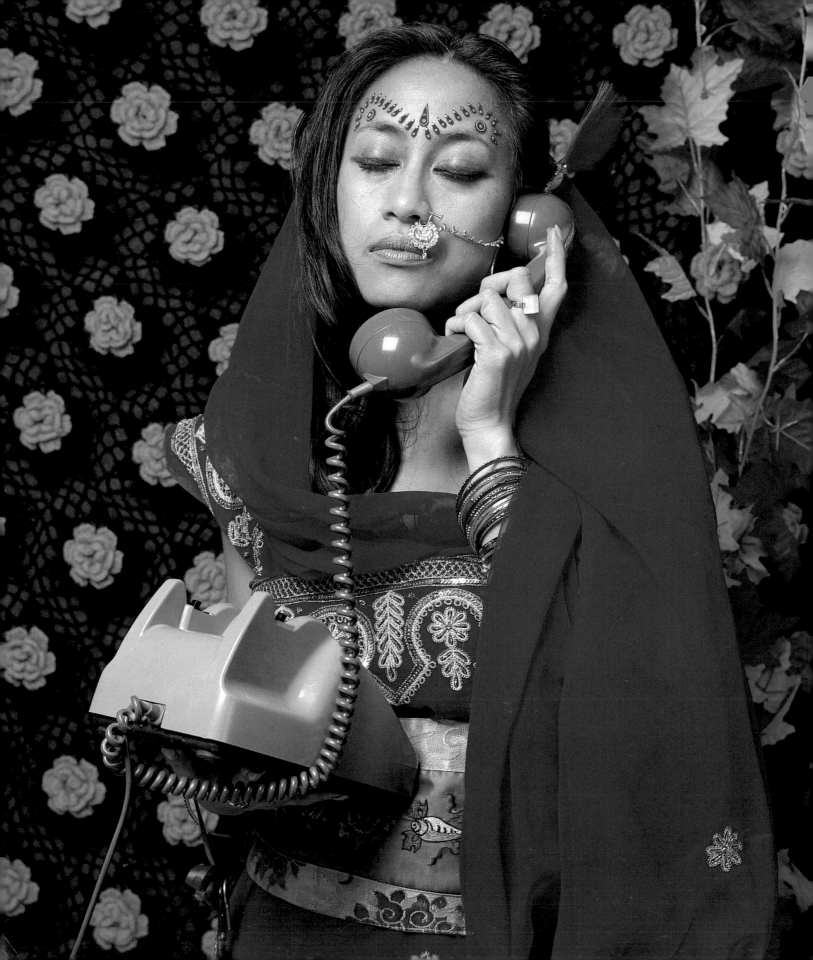

fashion victims. This 'Do-It-Yourself' approach to appearance has resulted in a cacophony of individual, often idiosyncratic expressions of self. In the process, every and any style or technique of human appearance modification has been enlisted – somewhere, by someone – in the cause of doing one's own thing.

Most remarkably, as discussed, this new, anything goes, approach to body decoration incorporates a massive new interest in and acceptance of many permanent techniques of body adornment. From Berlin to Buenos Aires, Sydney to San Francisco, especially (but not exclusively) among the young, tattooing and body piercing have become acceptable and normal to the extent that, at least in certain circles, not to have such permanent decorations is to be exceptional. Moreover, those in the avant-garde of this movement are often popstars, models, actors, athletes and other celebrities with enormous powers of influence in the media. That body piercings and tattoos are hip and aesthetically desirable is now constantly demonstrated in pop videos, advertisements, cinema, on fashion catwalks and television. Yet, only twenty or thirty years ago, to have tattoos or piercings (other than, and for women only, in the ear lobes) immediately and unconditionally set an individual beyond the limits of good taste and respectable society.

This prejudice against permanent body decoration has a long and fascinating history – fascinating because (ironically) Western, European civilization has its own roots firmly embedded in cultures that practised tattooing. The oldest surviving human body, that of the Iceman, preserved in the Italian Alps for some five thousand years, has thirteen small tattoos. The Egyptians, ancient Greeks and Romans used tattooing, and it is now widely accepted that at least some Anglo-Saxon and Celtic groups made it a key, even defining feature of their culture. It is now also thought that tattoo art was practised by some early Israelites and, subsequently, early Christians who, taking their lead from Saint Paul in Galatians 6:17 – 'I bear on my body the marks of Jesus' – had themselves tattooed with various Christian symbols (a practice that continued at least through medieval times for Christian pilgrims on reaching the Holy Land).

Despite all this, however, our Western prejudice against permanent body decoration has Judeo-Christian foundations. The 'Holiness Code' of Leviticus states, 'You shall not gash yourselves in mourning for the dead; you shall not tattoo yourselves'. Constantine, the first Christian emperor of Rome, prohibited tattooing (specifically, on the faces of criminals and

IN THE POSTMODERN ERA,
appearance and identity are sampled and mixed from divergent, often deliberately contrary sources. Instead of standardizing identity, and its signifier appearance, global culture increasingly celebrates pluralism and the unexpected. *opposite* Joan

slaves) on the grounds that, as we are fashioned in God's image, it is sacrilege to modify such a divine creation.

Yet, Christian pilgrims in the Holy Land and, according to some sources, throughout Europe, seem to have been unaffected by this line of reasoning. The really significant factor in the West's prejudice against permanent adornments came not with religion but with that dramatic shift in world view brought about by the Renaissance. Specifically, as European culture embraced that passion for constant change and progress that lay at the heart of Modernism, any permanent alteration of appearance became problematic. If this were not enough to set Western culture against permanent body decoration, first the Age of Exploration and then that of colonization sharpened the Western definition of civilization by contrasting it with savages who delighted in such barbaric practices as tattooing, scarification and piercing.

Yet, despite all this, tattooing persisted and even thrived within certain subgroups of Western society. However, despite the occasional fad among aristocrats for tattooing (for example, in Britain in the 19th century), these subgroups – sailors being the best known – were principally working-class. Up until the extraordinary pop culture revolution that occurred in the second half of the 20th century, good taste in all matters was always defined by the upper classes and so it is hardly surprising that tattooing remained stigmatized in respectable society.

So long-standing and entrenched was the West's classification of tattoos and other forms of permanent body decoration as barbaric and deviant, it is shocking to see how, in only a few decades, such a wide and socio-economically diverse cross section of people in Europe, Britain, North America, Australia and elsewhere has enthusiastically embraced them as legitimate, artistically sophisticated techniques of adornment. For this remarkable change in attitude to have taken root so widely and firmly, several profound cultural shifts had to take place more or less simultaneously within Western society.

The fanatical enthusiasm for change and progress that formed the cornerstone of the Western world view from the Renaissance onwards – propelling technological and other advances forward in the pursuit of the new and (therefore) improved – began to evaporate in the questioning times of the late 1960s. First the Hippies but then an ever-broader range of people came to feel that the brave new world of our future offered more to fear than to celebrate.

DIY, CUSTOM DESIGNS, developed in collaboration between client and tattooist, make each tattoo a unique conversation piece – a visual explication of self. *opposite* Anja, with the Mexican bingo card tattoos on her calves that she designed

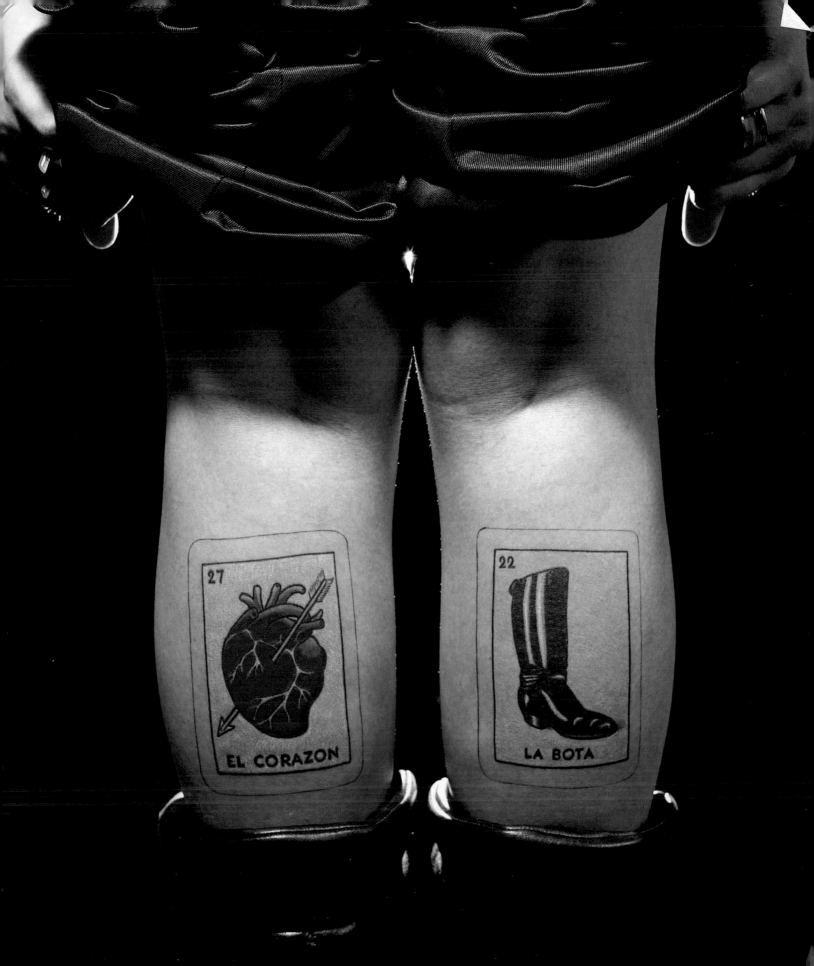

Entering the Postmodern era, opinions of change themselves began to change. Whereas most people had taken for granted the desirability of constant change and innovation, an influential minority (if not actually a majority) now started to crave stability in the face of a pace of change that increasingly seemed out of control. Taken together with premonitions of environmental and other disasters ahead, and the Generation Xers' realization that they (unlike the Baby Boomers) would be lucky to maintain, let alone surpass, the economic standards of their parents, a new world view emerged that feared transience and valued permanence.

Accordingly (body style always a particularly sensitive barometer of changing attitudes), consumers lost interest in a fashion industry focused exclusively on producing a neverending string of here-today-gone-tomorrow new looks and demanded instead (and got) a clothing industry more geared to the production of timeless classics, which could be worn from one year to the next and which advertised that the wearer was not a fickle fashion victim. This shift from fashion to classic personal style occurred in all spheres of appearance: shades of cosmetics, or hairstyles, that previously would have been systematically changed to comply with a new look fashion direction might now be proudly, defiantly maintained year after year as part of a consistent, unchanging statement of personal identity. At its most profound, however, this change in our attitude towards change brought about a dramatic and widespread reassessment of the permanent body decorations of tattooing and piercing. Suddenly, an adornment that lasts a lifetime seemed desirable rather than detrimental – a mechanism for symbolically resisting the whirlwinds of impermanence seen to threaten security; a device for demonstrating personal steadfastness in a world eroded by caprice.

On his return from the Pacific in 1773, the British explorer Captain Tobias Furneaux brought back to Britain a native from the island of Raiatea in the South Pacific (near Tahiti). Particularly because of his tattoos, Mai – or 'Omai' as he was mistakenly called – became one of the most famous inhabitants of London, and his example set a trend for the commercial exhibition of a considerable number of tattooed, pierced and scarred savages. While ever-popular, intriguing and fascinating, such individuals were never truly respected – their permanent body decorations a symbol of their inferior, primitive culture and proof of the higher state of Western civilization.

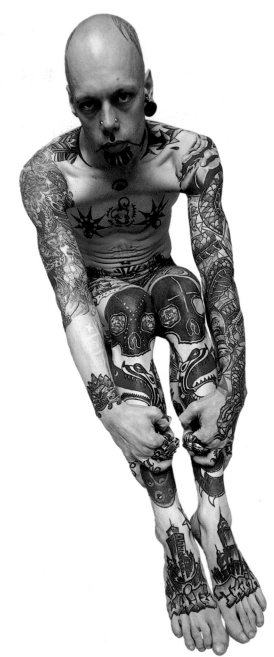

FOR THE COMMITTED
body decoration enthusiast there are seemingly no limits to the possibilities of self-expression. As mainstream acceptance of tattooing and piercing grows, ever more extreme looks are created. *above* Dave, body decoration artist at Tusk Tattoo & Body Piercing; *opposite* Lucky Diamond Rich, the world's most tattooed man. His skin has been 'coloured in' with tattoos (even inside his ears and nose) and now white designs are being overlaid

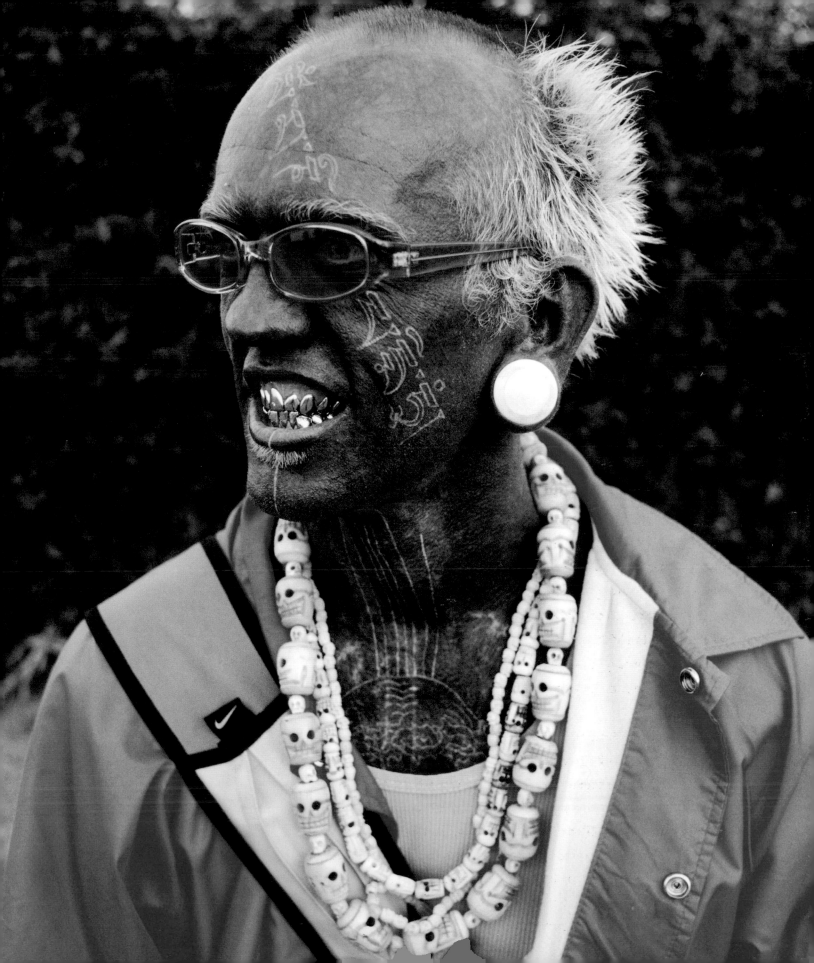

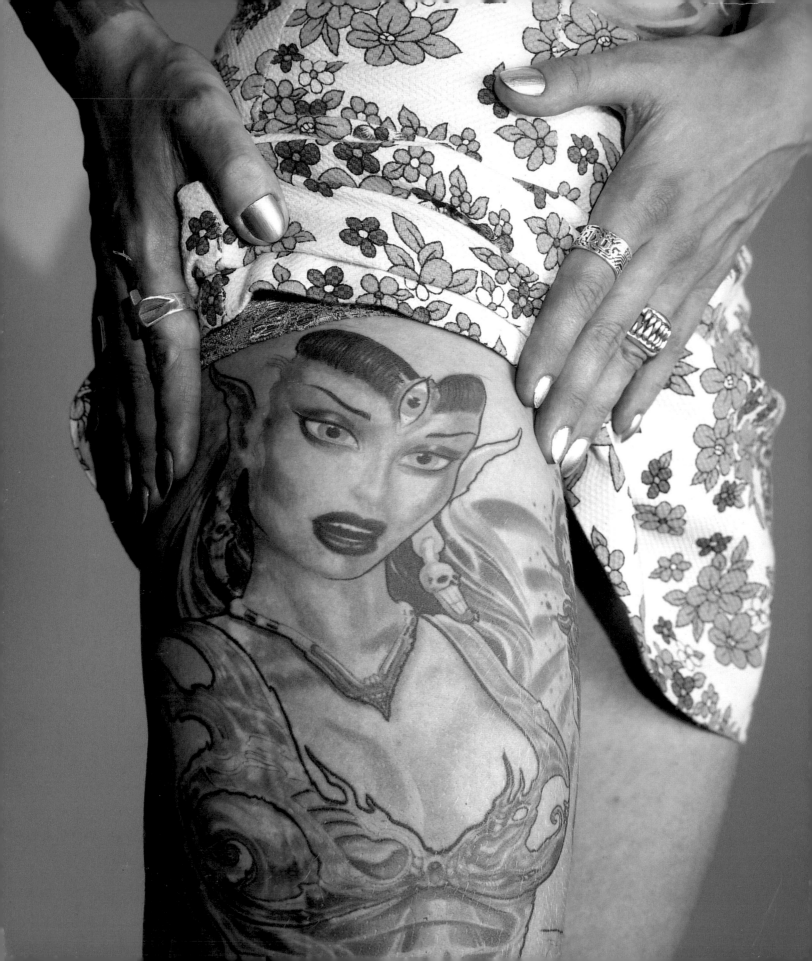

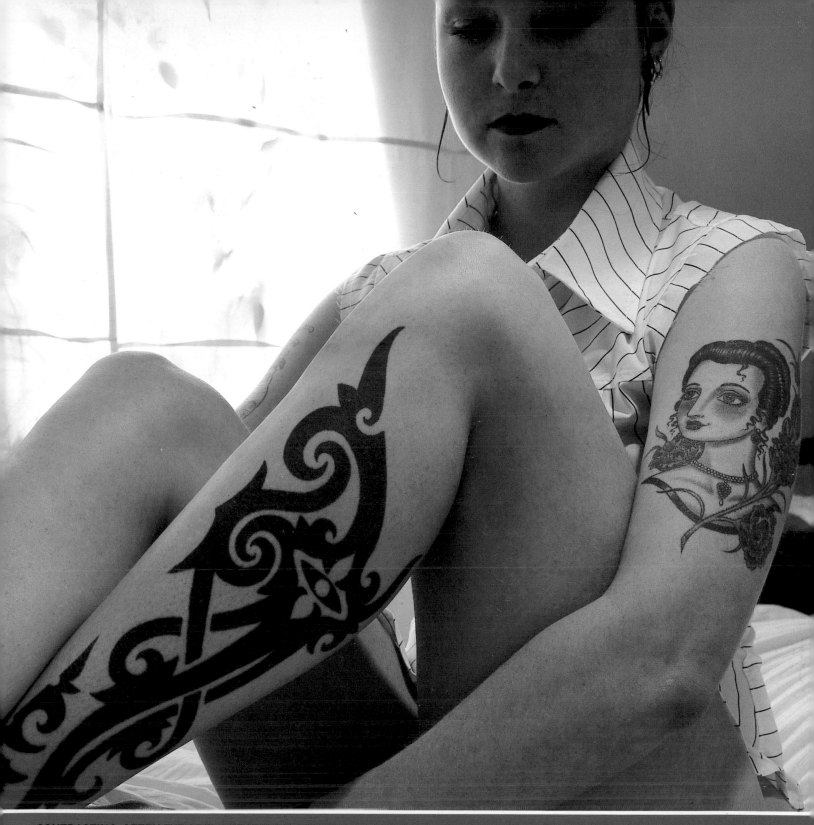

CONTRASTING, OFTEN EVEN DELIBERATELY CLASHING,
in today's supermarket of style clothing and body decoration become adjectives
in a complex, idiosyncratic statement of personal philosophy, values and dreams.
opposite D-Monica, custom leg tattoo, fine line freestyle by Claudia at House of
Tattoos; *above* Jannetje, Borneo Iban Tribal-style leg-piece by Jeroen Franken
and contrasting portrait of her mother by Chris Conn at Temple Tattoo

As discussed in 'The Exotic Body', the Hippies, the Punks and the Modern Primitives introduced (or, arguably, reflected) a growing respect for traditional – especially tribal – ways of life. With this respect came a new appreciation of many of the body decorations found among such peoples – their jewelry and hairstyles and also, significantly, their tattoos and piercings. Once proof of tribal peoples' barbarism, such permanent decorations are now increasingly seen as exemplary achievements of body art and symbols of a pre-industrial state of grace from which the West – ever-more out of control and spiritually impoverished – could learn something. We have, in other words, come a very long way from the time when the exhibition of the likes of Omai seemed to demonstrate the superiority of Western civilization. Indeed, the implication seems clear that a substantial number of people now see the cultures of tribal peoples as superior to their own, the most visible evidence of which is the extraordinary popularity of permanent Tribal and Primitive techniques and styles of body decoration.

Perhaps, given time, what the 20th century will be most remembered for is its unique democratization of culture – the small c in this word one of the most remarkable achievements of any era. The century began, like all others before it, with the definition of good taste and Culture firmly in the hands of the upper orders. But the 1920s saw how creations like jazz and tango, which were born on the wrong side of the tracks, could captivate the elite. Then, after World War II, the predominantly middle-class and university-educated Beats in America and the Left Bank Bohemians of Paris began an outright inversion of the sociocultural order during which good taste, superior style and sublime culture were seen to bubble up from the working class and the poor inhabitants of urban ghettos. What began as a minority fetish for anything and everything from the wrong side of the tracks, within just a few decades became a principal structural feature of our contemporary culture.

Most significantly, what bubbles up from the lower social strata is increasingly perceived as possessing an authenticity that High Culture is incapable of delivering. Within our contemporary 'twilight of the real' (to use Neville Wakefield's telling phrase) the crisis of authenticity is seen as the key problem, by a wide range of cultural theorists. It is hardly surprising, therefore (yet, nevertheless astonishing in historical terms), to see the speed with which anything perceived as real by virtue of its impoverished street cred roots has been transformed from

SEEN AS ABERRANT, EVEN DEGENERATE, only a generation ago, tattoos today are increasingly viewed as a normal part of personal expression. Is the time fast approaching when those without a distinctive tattoo or piercing will be classed as naked and unrespectable? *opposite* Yazzamin's chest tattoo is a continuing project – starting life as a small ladybird it is being expanded by Amar and Marty at Tattoo Peter

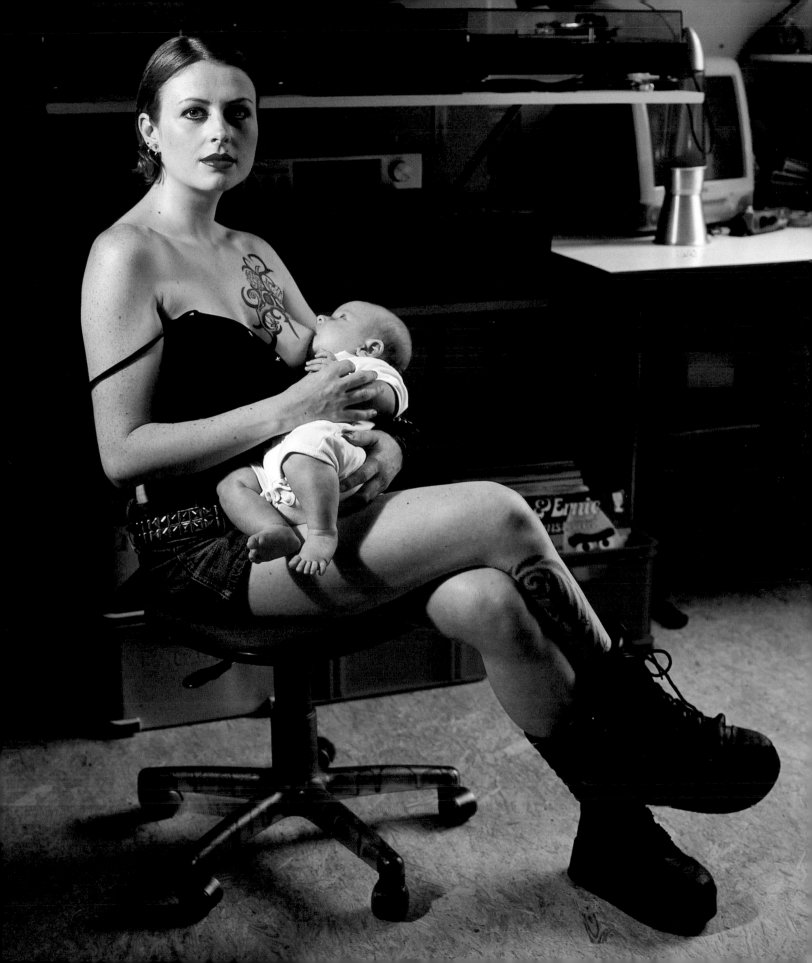

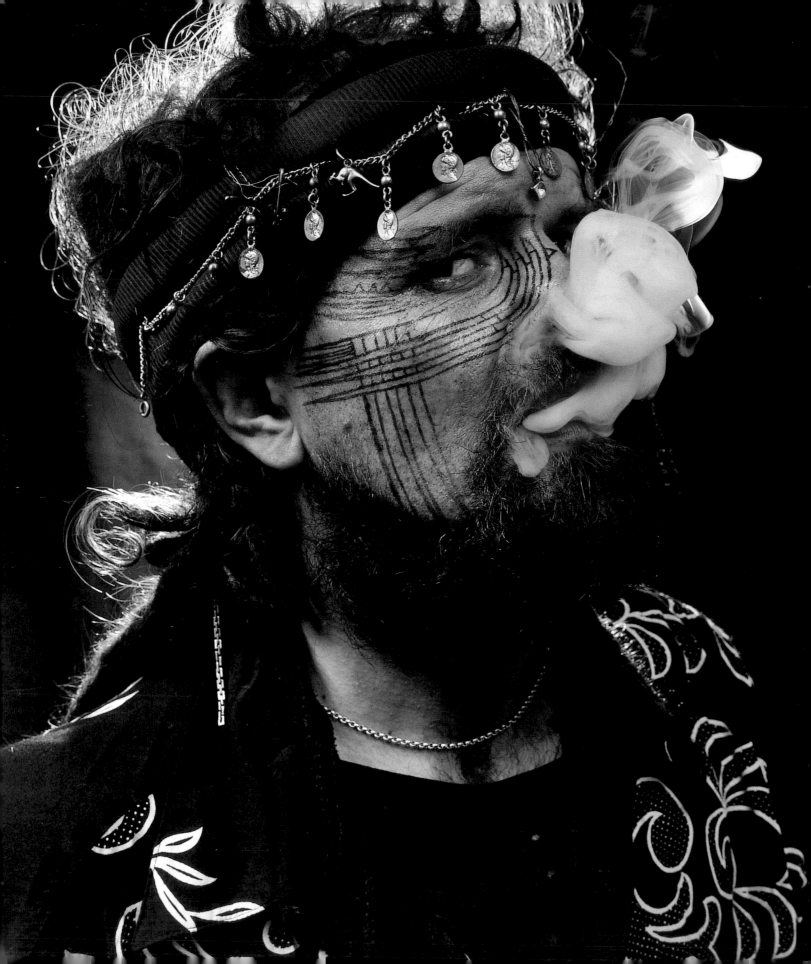

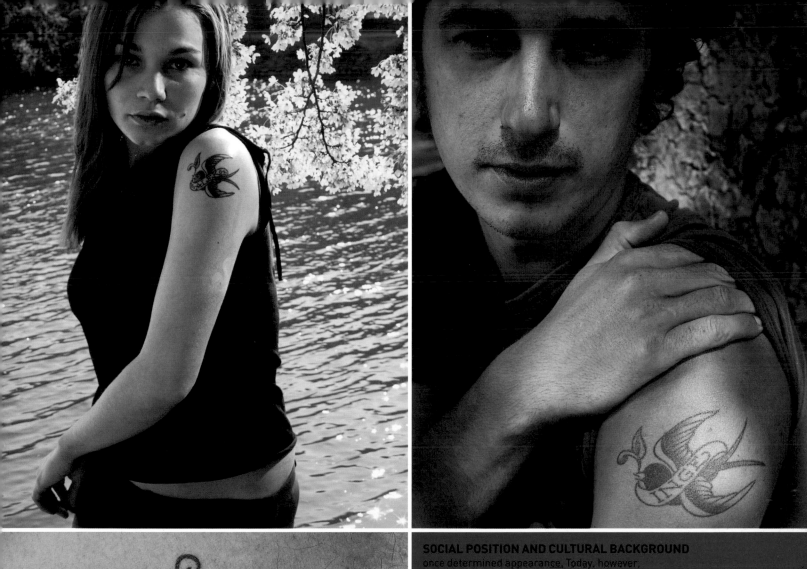

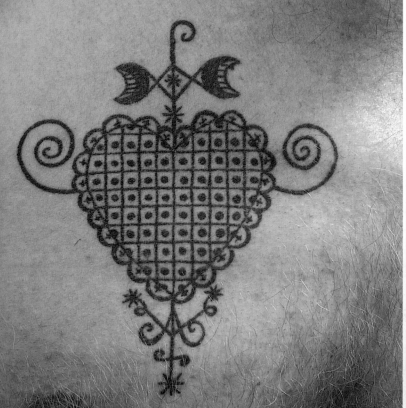

SOCIAL POSITION AND CULTURAL BACKGROUND

once determined appearance. Today, however, we reach out to others, establish relationships and position ourselves in the universe by means of a self-customized appearance style that signals 'I am here'. To fail to be distinctive is to disappear socially as well as visually. *opposite* Jan Dominic with Neo Tribal-style face paint he wears daily; *above* Alex and Inge with Folk-style tattoos of each other's names, which were made after their second date to mark their commitment to the relationship; *left* Mark's distinctive voodoo heart tattoo

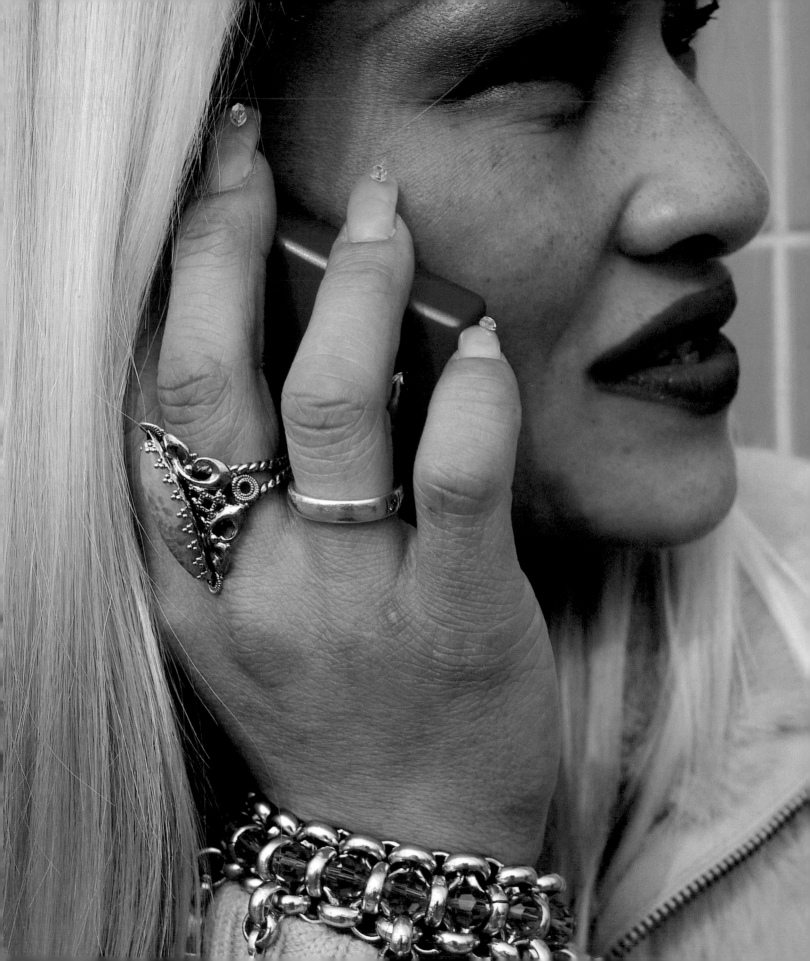

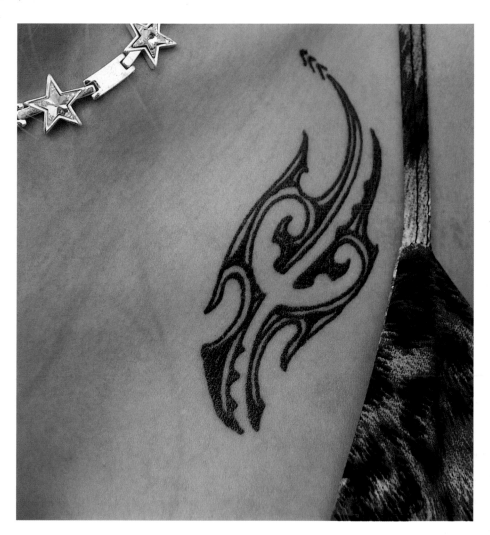

naff to pukka; from embarrassment to treasure, from lead to gold. It is for this
reason that the fashion world has come to scour (and rip off) streetstyle for inspiration. However, when, for example, Marlon Brando's black leather Perfecto-style
jacket (as worn in *The Wild One*) becomes an upmarket fashionalized garment
that anyone with enough money can purchase, something is inevitably lost in the
translation – namely, the very aura of authenticity which gave the original
garment its 'real' value.

But a tattoo...now that has potential. As we noted earlier, one of the reasons
for the inhibition of mainstream acceptance of tattooing was its long-term
associations with the lower classes. Now that such prejudice has been turned
on its head, however, the tattoo gains rather than loses cultural value from
this association. Even more than this, the permanence of tattoos coupled
with the pain involved in acquiring them – that their cost, in other words, is
not merely financial – allows them to retain a great deal of their original

authenticity. In the age of replicants and simulations, the prick of the tattooist's needle signifies – so it is hoped – commitment, steadfastness and, crucially, the authenticity of a life untainted by the discreet but synthetic charms of the bourgeoisie.

And so it has come to pass that two permanent forms of adornment – tattooing and piercing – occupy an increasingly respected place within our expanding repertoire of body decoration techniques and are respected, in particular, for their demonstration of constancy and commitment; their symbolic links to primitive and proletarian credibility. It is the juxtaposition of this dramatic increase in the acceptance of permanent body adornment with a more liberated, more personally creative, post-fashion approach to the stylistic possibilities of all forms of body decoration that makes the current situation so unprecedented and exciting.

There are still some techniques of decoration (for example scarification) that have not, at least so far, crossed over from the extreme fringes of experimentation to the mainstream. It is also true – amazingly, after decades heralding a unisex revolution, and the possibilities raised by Punks, New Romantics and Goths – that make-up, nail art and various hairstyles continue to be taboo for real men. Finally, the workplace continues to discourage and prohibit a great deal of experimentation with new appearance styles that so many people now see as a vital part of their expression of personal identity. (This conflict will soon become critical and conservative employers are certain to lose in time.)

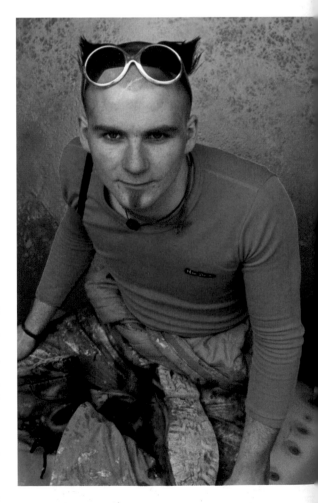

Yet even when these restrictions are factored in, the contemporary world's approach to the decoration and transformation of the body can only be described as extraordinary; all the more so because of the phenomenal speed with which this international revolution has taken place. Only thirty years ago if you had predicted that normal, average, mainstream men and women would want a tattoo or a piercing, everyone would have laughed. Likewise, if you had argued that fashion would lose its dictatorial power no one would have taken you seriously. Yet this – and much more – is exactly what has happened: with individual choice and personal creativity in matters of appearance not only untethered, but a necessary, fundamental part of life in the 21st century.

A woman now buys a new lipstick or eyeshadow because the colour suits her rather than, as previously, because a fashion magazine told her which shades are currently in. Likewise, someone who wants a tattoo, instead of simply

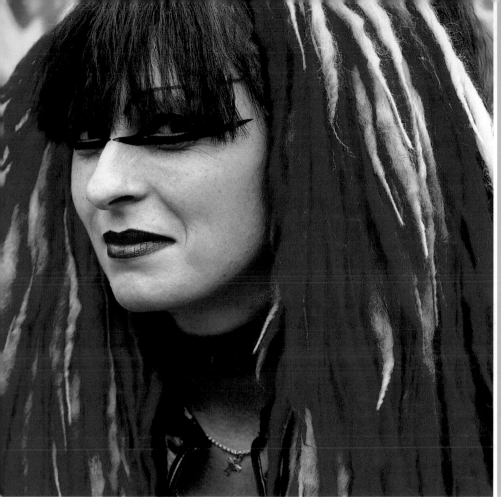

A DYNAMIC, SELF-CONSTRUCTED MATRIX
of values, beliefs and lifestyle options, identity is no longer determined by background, geography, social position or profession. Difficult, often impossible to put into words, the most precise and resonant articulation of identity is that of personal presentation of self, appearance. Saying much more than simply 'I am rich' or 'I am fashionable', appearance uses the medium of the superficial to project deeply held beliefs. *clockwise from opposite* Jason, Lisa, Grace and Denise

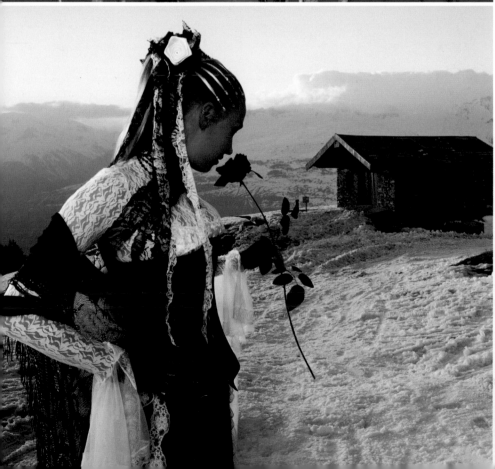

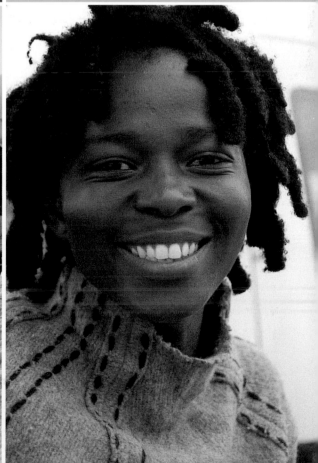

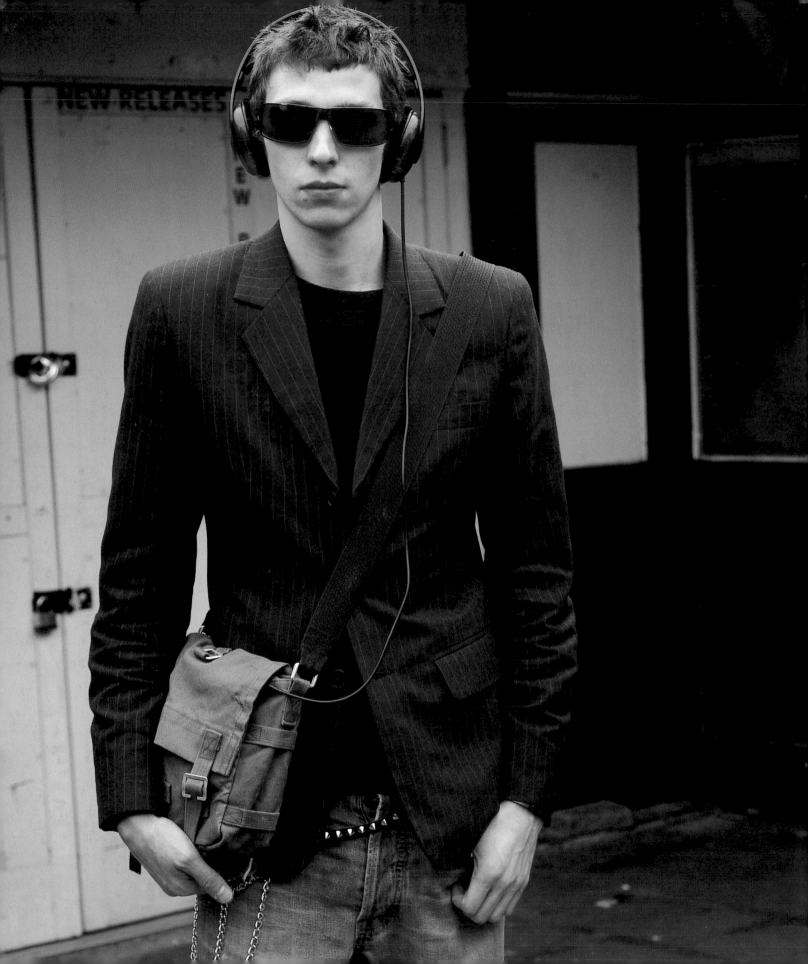

selecting a pierced heart or bluebird from a selection of ageing flash drawings, will come up with his or her own ideas, which will be developed in collaboration with the tattooist. In both instances (and the same is true in hairstyling, nail art, jewelry, piercing, accessories and clothing) the individual creatively engages in the construction of his or her unique, visual identity.

Such Do-It-Yourself styling takes a lot of time and energy, but it is not just narcissism that causes us to expend such effort. In every era of human history body decoration and dress have served vital, arguably critical purposes. For traditional peoples, they demarcated group boundaries and functioned as a symbol of cultural continuity. In the modern era, in the form of fashion – a kind of timekeeping device – they gave tangible proof of change and progress. In the present era body decoration and dress are elucidating an invaluable vocabulary of personal identity.

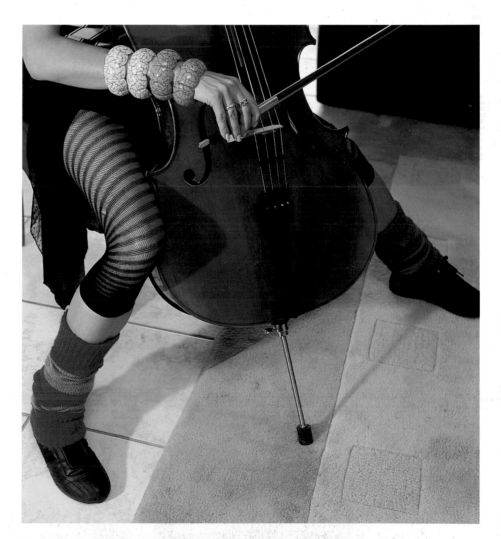

TODAY, EVERYONE IS A STYLIST,
creating his or her own look; marketing themselves. The sheer number of stylistic options available has widened our choices in personal appearance as never before. *opposite* James; *right* Tory

Only a generation or two ago a person's identity was principally defined by the world they were born into – their class, nationality, religion, race, ethnic background and so forth. In this world 'Who are you?' was a simple question with simple verbal answers. In the current age, however, 'Who are you?' is both more subtle and problematic. We want others to have a complex, multifaceted understanding of us that goes beyond where we came from and what we do for a living. We want – no, we need – to express all those values, beliefs and dreams that triangulate 'where we are at'. Unfortunately (as is all too evident in any text-only lonely hearts ad) verbal language is not usually up to this task, and so, like our most distant ancestors, we resort to that more symbolic, resonant and multifarious language of visual style – our choices of furniture, car, garden, pets or cuisine all becoming part of a statement about ourselves. But it is our choice of appearance style – so intimate yet portable, omnipresent and demanding of a special level of personal commitment – that serves as our ultimate tool for marketing and advertising ourselves. To find others on our particular wave-length – People Like Us – we must devise a look that succeeds in translating our respective personalities and visions into the ever-expanding vocabulary of clothing and body decoration. To fail to use this tool effectively – to fail to project our inner selves in a way that marks us out and differentiates us from the amorphous mass our global culture has become – is to remain isolated and invisible. In a sense, to cease to be. For as Descartes might have put it, had he lived in the 21st century, 'I look distinctive – like me – therefore I am.'

A SINGLE GLANCE IS ALL IT TAKES
to evaluate astounding amounts of data. Once upon a time people met other people by means of an introduction. Today people meet – or choose not to – on the basis of appearance. Does your appearance say what you want it to say about you? *opposite* Sherwin

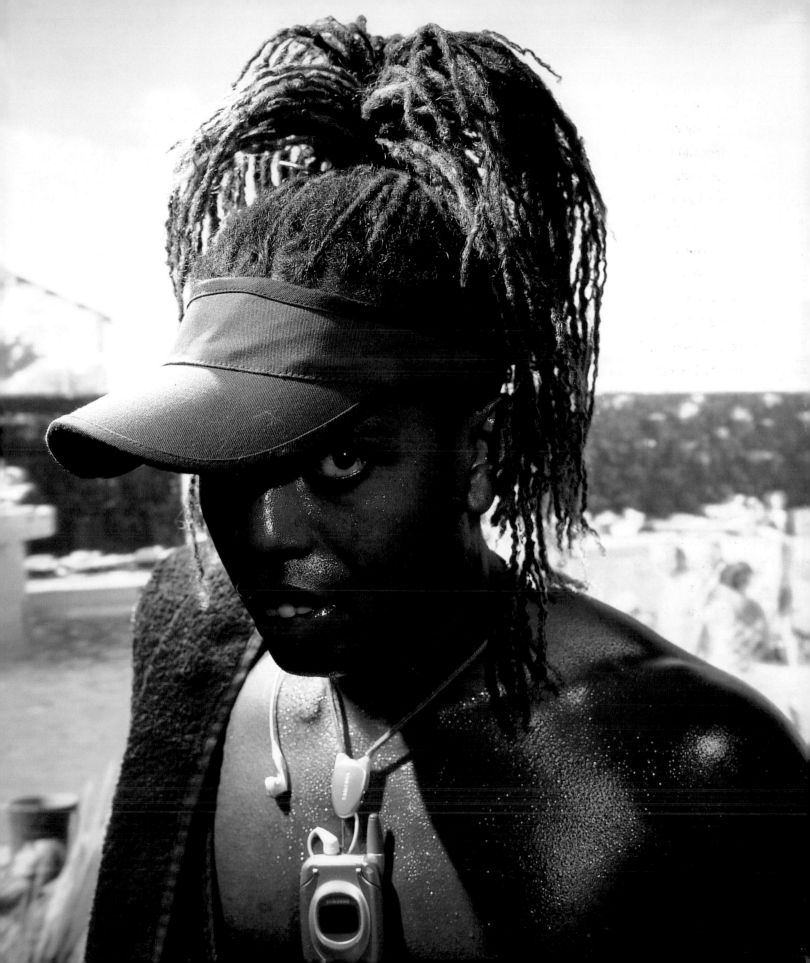

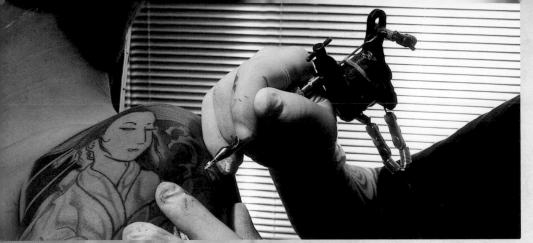

PRACTICAL ADVICE ON GETTING A TATTOO

PATIENCE AND CHOICE

Getting a tattoo is a special experience and should never be hurried. Be prepared to take all the time you need to find the right design and the right tattooist, and to wait for an appointment. Never choose to have a tattoo done because your friends (or a celebrity) have done it. Never do it unless you are 100 per cent certain that the choice is entirely yours. There should be no emulation or competition in tattooing. Consider it to be one of the most personal choices you will ever make.

Betti Marenko by Mrs Love>in.sect.corp™

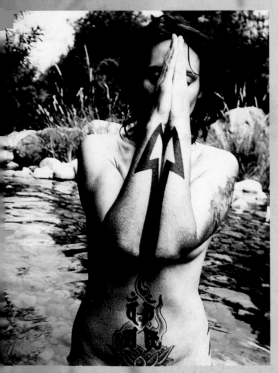

PAIN

A few myths to dispel: getting tattooed is not as painful as many suspect, although it may be uncomfortable, depending on its placement on the body. Some parts of the body may be naturally more sensitive than others (i.e. any 'bony' area, compared to any 'fleshy' area). Having said that, there is no body part 'better' than any other for a tattoo. Ultimately it depends on both individual taste and the extent to which you are willing to be public with your tattoo, although reputable tattooists will refuse to do hands or faces. Irrational fear is the worst pain-trigger of all. Reaction to pain varies enormously from one individual to the next. Hence, you must be aware of your own pain threshold and be adequately prepared. If you know you are prone to fainting at the sight of needles or blood you may want to take some precautions since tattooing includes both of these. However, this does NOT mean taking drugs of any sort, including alcohol, since by altering your perception these will make the experience even worse, rather than helping you to relax. Instead, aim to be in a good mood. Devote some time to preparing yourself and your body for this unique experience. Acknowledge pain as a new sensation to feel, rather than something to fear and avoid. Pain comes in waves. Try to 'surf' them. The more accepting you are of pain, the more you will be able to embrace it, become one with it and feel elation rather than distress. Tattooing is very much a collaborative process between you and your tattooist. He or she knows which parts of the body are bound to be more uncomfortable and will have the expertise to put you at ease. Listen carefully to his or her advice on the matter and trust it.

AFTERCARE

Always follow your tattooist's recommendations. Generally a new tattoo should be bandaged for at least one hour and for no longer than eight hours. Do not rebandage it. Wash it gently in warm running water and mild soap after removing the bandage. Do not scrub. Do not use a washcloth. Make sure you get all blood, products and ointments off the tattoo. Pat dry with a clean towel, or better, whenever possible, allow it to air dry. Apply a small amount of unscented dye-free quality moisturizer, enough to prevent your tattoo from drying out. Gently rub it in, at least twice a day until the tattoo has healed (approximately nine to fourteen days). Do not pick or scratch any scabs. Do not swim (in either salt or chlorinated water), sunbathe or soak the tattooed area. Do keep it clean and free from dust, paint, cement and oil (including sun oil). Most importantly: do not scratch! Your tattoo will itch as it heals, but you must allow the scabs to flake off in their own time. Wear loose clothing that allows your tattoo to breathe, but does not rub against it. If you suspect the tattoo is becoming infected, inform the tattooist and consult a doctor. The healing process depends on your own care and responsibility. Be kind to yourself and always follow your tattooist's instructions.

SAFETY

Tattooing is perfectly safe if proper sterilization and infection control standards are followed: anything that comes in contact with blood or bodily fluids must either be disposed of (single-use)[1] or sterilized (autoclaved).[2] Look carefully at the appearance of the studio and ask questions. Is the studio clean and professional-looking? Does it have a licence from the local Department of Health? Any health-service environment, including a tattooing studio, in which contact with blood and bodily fluids is possible, must have certification. Is there an autoclave? Are the needles and other items single-use? What kind of disinfectants are used? A professional and responsible studio takes pride in its health and safety procedures and will happily answer all your questions.

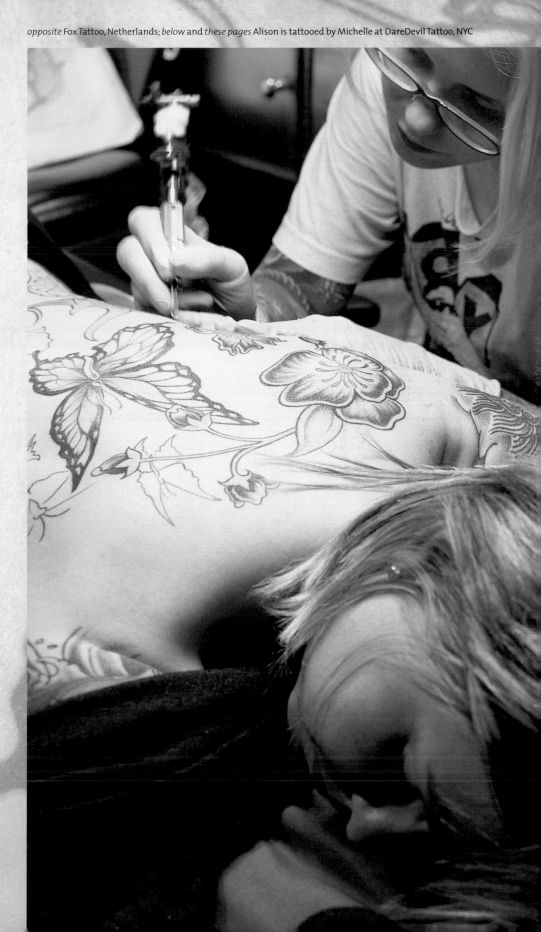

RELIABILITY

Check the studio and the staff. Are they polite and presentable? Do you feel comfortable there? A tattoo artist should be helpful, answer your questions honestly and put you at ease. Check that he or she is a member of any professional organizations. Reputable tattooists are devoted to maintaining high standards of tattooing, to celebrating it as an art form and to protecting the industry. Ask how long they have been tattooing and have a look at photos of their work, flash drawings and other art. A good artist's work is always his or her best advertisement! Ask about their training and their drawing skills. If you go for custom work you want to choose an artist you feel comfortable with and who will collaborate with you in drawing up the perfect tattoo that fits your body and your vision.

COST

The cost should never dictate the choice of artist or design. Think how many other purchases you are likely to make in a lifetime that will be with you, actually becoming you, forever. In fact, cost should be a minor factor in your decision. If you take price as a governing criteria it is better to wait and avoid disappointment. You will have the tattoo a lot longer than the tattooist will have the money and a tattoo that you are happy with is priceless.

A FINAL WORD OF ADVICE

Tattoos are not meant for everyone. Getting a tattoo is a personal decision that you will live with for the rest of your life, so make sure you research your design well and then find a good artist whom you trust to do the work. Go and see as many artists as you like. It is your tattoo. It is your body. It is forever.

[1] Every set of needles used to apply a tattoo should be brand new, including the bars and grommets, individually packaged, sealed, and autoclaved.
[2] An autoclave is a heat/steam/pressure unit that is the only acceptable way to sterilize things in a tattoo studio. When used properly it will kill all known organisms, including their spores.

PRACTICAL ADVICE ON GETTING A PIERCING

PREPARING YOUR BODY

When planning a piercing consider your current state of health. If your immune system is weakened by illness, drugs, alcohol, or even lack of sleep, the potential for infection and/or rejection of body jewelry increases. Eat well, as you need to maintain safe blood-sugar levels. Do not have a piercing on an empty stomach as you may faint, but do not eat a big meal immediately before either. Allow one to two hours between your meal and your appointment. Your body's endorphin response may lead to unease when combined with a full stomach. Do not use alcohol, drugs or caffeine for twenty-four hours prior to and for several hours after the piercing as these may increase bleeding, or cause dizziness and vomiting.

YOUR PIERCING APPOINTMENT

Visit several piercing studios and observe the work area. Is it kept in a clean and sanitary condition? Does it have good lighting? Is there an autoclave? Ask to see the sterilization equipment. If the piercer refuses to discuss cleanliness and infection control, go somewhere else. If they are reputable they will take pride in being helpful and showing you around.

IMMEDIATELY BEFORE PIERCING

The piercer must wash and dry his or her hands and wear latex gloves. Gloves must be worn at all times during the piercing procedure. If any other object is touched (such as a phone), the piercer must wear new gloves.

Never accept a piercing done with a piercing gun as this cannot be properly sterilized. Body piercing should be done ONLY with a new, sterile needle in order to minimize risk of exposure to the HIV/AIDS and Hepatitis B viruses. Jewelry must be made of a non-corrosive metal, such as surgical stainless steel, niobium, titanium or solid fourteen-carat gold. Gold-plated jewelry should not be used.

Before piercing you should be given a consent form. If you are a minor you will need a signed consent form from your parents.[1] Remember that not all piercings suit all bodies. Your piercer can advise on how to choose the piercing best suited to your body shape.

AFTERCARE

Always wash your hands before touching the piercing. Remove any dressing after one to two hours and do not reapply, unless you are in a very dirty/dusty environment. Clean your piercing two to four times daily with a mild, undyed, unfragranced, non-creamy soap.[2] Gently remove all dry matter (lymph fluid and dead skin cells) from the jewelry before moving it, or it will scratch and reopen your piercing. Whenever possible air dry. Avoid any contact with foreign bodily fluid to the area (sweat, blood, saliva, etc.). Try not to catch your piercing accidentally. Do not wear anything that rubs against it. Be careful if using a swimming pool during healing as bacteria and poor quality water may cause infection.[3] Be aware that common skincare products may contain irritant components.

Do not remove the jewelry until well after the piercing is completely healed. Once healed, a piercing is permanent. Removal of jewelry will cause the hole to shrink, and jewelry re-insertion will need a gentle stretching beforehand. Failure to clean your piercing may lead to infection.

DO USE

Salt water is the least reactive and most effective cleaning solution (1/4 teaspoon of salt to one cup of clean water).[4] Also good are seawater and your own urine. Urine is a sterile cleaning agent as the uric acid it contains kills bacteria without hindering the formation of new cells.

Essential oil of lavender is a natural antibiotic and a few drops may be added to a salt water solution. All immune system boosters (vitamin C, echinacea, ginseng and garlic) will speed healing. During the healing period your piercing is the most vulnerable part of your body, so it will be affected by a low immune system, physical and emotional stress, hormone changes and PMS, etc. The better you treat your body by eating well, sleeping enough and avoiding stress, drugs and alcohol, the faster your piercing will heal. A zinc supplement at the beginning will also help. Vitamin E at the end of the healing period helps prevent excess scarring.

AVOID

Alcohol and hydrogen peroxide are far too harsh and can destroy new healing tissue. Antibiotic ointments, especially on the genitals, septum, nostrils and near eyes or inner lips are not necessary unless treating infection and directed by a doctor.[5] Perfumed, dyed or cream soaps, make-up, perfume and hair products may contain irritants. Plasters create an ideal thriving place for bacteria. Avoid holding a public telephone against a newly pierced ear. Finally, avoid excessive handling and overcleaning.

IN CASE OF INFECTION

The body recognizes a new piercing as if it were a sliver, thus some discharge and a little redness are normal. However, if signs of infection are present (increased redness, tenderness, heat, swelling) antibiotics may be necessary. See your

this page tummy button piercing, Dave at Tusk, London *opposite* piercing jewelry *opposite far right* multiple ear piercings

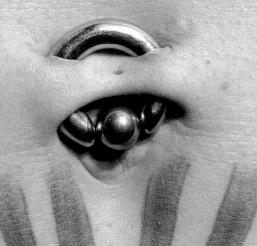

piercer and seek medical treatment. In particular, be careful of infection in nasal piercings as this may cause serious complications. If you are allergic to the jewelry, the skin around the piercing will look as if it is pulling away – have jewelry replaced with more compatible materials.

HEALING TIMES

All body piercings require diligent care and time to heal, depending on their placement. Humans have been healing piercings for thousands of years without antibiotics or soap. Your body knows how to heal a piercing. If you keep your piercing clean and take good care of your body you will heal fast and well.

Ear lobe	6 to 8 weeks
Ear cartilage	4 months to 1 year
Eyebrow	6 to 8 weeks
Nostril	2 to 4 months
Nasal septum	6 to 8 months
Nasal bridge	8 to 10 weeks
Tongue	4 weeks
Lip	2 to 3 months
Nipple	3 to 6 months
Navel	4 months to 1 year
Female genitals	4 to 10 weeks
Male genitals	4 weeks to 6 months

ORAL

Piercings inside the mouth (i.e. the tongue, the inside of labret, lip and cheek) are usually kept clean by saliva. In addition, rinse your mouth with salt water or alcohol-free mouthwash,[6] several times each day, especially after eating, drinking and smoking. To reduce initial swelling of the tongue suck on ice cubes. Eat soft food. Avoid excessive talking, sharing drinks and oral sex. Smoking, spicy foods, tomato juice, spirits and citrus juices will sting. Once the swelling has gone the jewelry can be downsized.

GENITALS

Genital piercings (both female and male) heal fast and successfully thanks to the good blood supply in the area. For this reason they may also bleed a little more than others. Avoid all sexual activity for two weeks – do not get too playful for the first month to avoid bruising, tearing or hurting the piercing. Use a condom or dental dam for a few weeks afterwards as you may risk infection (even in monogamous relationships). Male genital piercings are cleaned internally every time you urinate, so drinking plenty of water helps.

STRETCHING

Stretching means to enlarge a piercing by gradually inserting bigger jewelry. The effect is to turn the piercing from semi-permanent (for the first twelve to eighteen months a piercing will close rapidly if jewelry is not worn) to permanent. If you decide to go for stretching, it is important to be extra-patient, proceed slowly and respect healing times at all stages. Rushing the process will only cause problems later on. Each individual is different and the amount of time required between stretches can vary. However, it is advisable to wait at least six weeks between one stretching and the next and, as always, to seek the advice of a professional on whether or not stretching is appropriate to a particular piercing.

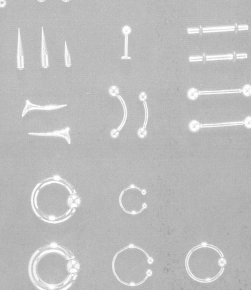

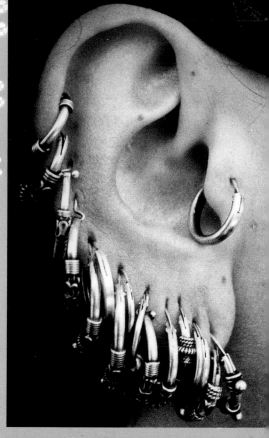

A FINAL WORD ON PIERCING

Getting pierced demands total trust in your piercer and in yourself. The rewards can be high, revealing a great deal not only about your body but about your capacity to be vulnerable, to trust and to conquer your fears (and not only the fear of needles). Because it creates an opening in the body, piercing is an experience in which exposure and strength converge in the here and now. For these reasons, and for many others as numerous as each individual, piercing has a strong ritualistic aspect, and is often seen as a tool of growth and self-understanding.

[1] Laws concerning piercing, including the age of consent, may vary.
[2] Glycerine anti-bacterial soaps eg. Neutrogena, Allenbury's and Pears; Tea Tree Soap; Dr Bronner's Baby Soap. Bactine antiseptic solution may be used.
[3] Vaseline or Neosporin may be dabbed through the hole to seal off the exposed tissue temporarily. After swimming clean immediately with salt water.
[4] Other products (active ingredient usually benzalkonium chloride) include: Bacitracin Zinc, Bactine (to dilute: 3 parts water to 1 part solution), Betadine (be careful as it will discolour gold jewelry), Hibiclens, Benzalkonium Chloride, Campho Phenique, and D-Alpha Vitamin E oil.
[5] For instance, Hibitane, Bactroban, Baciguent, Hibiclens (do not use for piercings above shoulders as it may cause deafness or blindness). Also, do not use Neosporin and Polysporin, as they contain petroleum products.
[6] Tech 2000, Biotene or Tea Tree Mouthwash

BIBLIOGRAPHY

Ahmed, S. and Stacey, J. (eds), *Thinking Through the Skin*, London and New York, 2001

Australian Museum, *Body Art*, Mosman, Australia, 2000

Barbieri, Gian Paolo, *Tahiti Tattoos*, Cologne, 1998

Batra, Sumita, *The Art of Mehndi*, London, 1999

Baudot, François, *A Century of Fashion*, London, 1999

Becker, Vivienne, *Ethnic Rich: Swarovski Celebrates Ethnic Jewellery*, Vienna, 1996

Beckwith, Carol and Angela Fisher, *African Ark*, London, 1992 (3rd edn)

Benthien, C., *Skin: On the Cultural Border Between Self and the World*, New York, 2002

Bohannan, Paul, 'Beauty and Scarification Amongst the Tiv' in Arnold Rubin (ed.), *Marks of Civilization*, Los Angeles, 1988, pp. 77–82

Boucher, François, *A History of Costume in the West*, London, 1987

Brain, Robert, *The Decorated Body*, London, 1979

British Museum, *Masks and the Art of Expression*, New York, 1994

Burchett, George, *Memoirs of a Tattooist: From the Notes, Diaries and Letters of the Late 'King of Tattooists'*, London, 1958

Camphausen, Rufus C., *Return of the Tribal: A Celebration of Body Adornment*, Rochester, USA, 1997

Caplan, Jane (ed.), *Written on the Body: The Tattoo in European and American History*, London, 2000

Clarke, Pauline, *The Eye of the Needle*, Nuneaton, UK, 1994

Connor, S., *The Book of Skin*, London, 2004

Debord, Guy, *The Society of the Spectacle*, New York, 1995

Delio, Michelle, *Tattoo: The Exotic Art of Skin Decoration*, New York, 1993

DeMello, Margo, *Bodies of Inscription: A Cultural History of the Modern Tattoo Community*, Durham, USA, 2000

Dunbar, Andrew and Dean Lahn, *Body Piercing*, New York, 1998

Durfee, Dale, *Tattoo*, New York, 2000

Dwyer, Jane Powell (ed.), *The Cashinahua of Eastern Peru*, Boston, 1975

Ebensten, Hanns, *Pierced Hearts and True Love: The History of Tattooing*, London, 1953

Ebin, Victoria, *The Body Decorated*, London, 1979

Ebong, Ima (ed.), *Black Hair: Art, Style, and Culture*, New York, 2001

Faris, James C., *Nuba Personal Art*, London, 1972

Featherstone, M. (ed.), 'Body Modification', *Body & Society*, 5 (2-3) special issue, London, 1999

Fisher, Angela, *Africa Adorned*, London, 1987 (3rd edn)

Flugel, J. C., *The Psychology of Clothes*, London, 1971

Fontanel, Béatrice, *Support and Seduction: A History of Corsets and Bras*, New York, 1997

Galerie Ra, *Maskerade: Contemporary Masks by Fifty Artists*, Amsterdam, 2001

Gell, A., *Wrapping in Images: Tattooing in Polynesia*, Oxford, 1993

Gerard, Jim, *Celebrity Skin: Tattoos, Brands and Body Adornment of the Stars*, Hove, UK, 2001

Gilbert, Steve, *Tattoo History: A Source Book*, New York, 2000

Goffman, Erving, *The Presentation of Self in Everyday Life*, London, 1969

Gröning, Karl, *Decorated Skin: A World Survey of Body Art*, London, 1997

Hardy, D. E. (ed.), *Pierced Hearts and True Love: A Century of Drawings for Tattoos*, New York and Honolulu, 1995

Hardy, D. E. and 'Studio I' (eds), *L'Asino e la zebra: Origini e tendenze del tatuaggio contemporaneo*, Rome, 1985

Hewitt, K., *Mutilating the Body: Identity in Blood and Ink*, Bowling Green, USA, 1997

Howell, Georgina, *In Vogue: Six Decades of Fashion*, London, 1975

Jaguer, Jeff, *The Tattoo: A Pictorial History*, Horndean, UK, 1990

Jones, Dylan, *Haircults: Fifty Years of Styles and Cuts*, London, 1990

King, J. C. H. (ed.), *Human Image*, London, 2000

Kitamura, T. and Kitamura K. M., *Bushido: Legacies of the Japanese Tattoo*, Atglen, PA, USA, 2001

Klippensteen, Kate, *Ganguro Girls: The Japanese 'Black Face'*, Cologne, 2001

Krakow, Amy, *The Total Tattoo Book*, New York, 1994

Lautman, Victoria, *The New Tattoo*, New York, 1994

Lazi, Claudio and Catherine Grognard, *The Tattoo: Graffiti for the Soul*, London, 1994

Leuzinger, Elsy, *The Art of Black Africa*, Barcelona, 1985

Lévi-Strauss, Claude, *Structural Anthropology*, London, 1969

Lévi-Strauss, Claude, *Tristes tropiques*, Harmondsworth, UK, 1984

Lobenthal, Joel, *Radical Rags: Fashions of the Sixties*, New York, 1990

Mack, John (ed.), *Masks and the Art of Expression*, London, 1994

McCabe, M., *New York City Tattoo: The Oral History of an Urban Art*, Honolulu, 1997

McCabe, M., *Tattooing New York City: Style and Continuity in a Changing Art Form*, Atglen, PA, USA, 2001

McLaughlin, Terence, *The Gilded Lily*, London, 1972

McNab, Nan, *Body Bizarre Body Beautiful*, New York, 1999

Mercury, Maureen, *Pagan Fleshworks: The Alchemy of Body Modification*, Rochester, USA, 2000

Mertens, Alice and Joan Broster, *African Elegance*, London, 1974

Mifflin, Margot, *Bodies of Subversion: A Secret History of Women and Tattoo*, New York, 1997 (2nd edn)

Miller, Jean-Chris, *The Body Art Book*, New York, 1997

Morris, Desmond, *Bodywatching: A Field Guide to the Human Species*, London, 1987

Morris, Desmond, *The Naked Ape*, London, 1967

Mulvey, Kate and Melissa Richards, *Decades of Beauty: The Changing Image of Women 1890s – 1990s*, London, 1998

Musafar, Fakir, *Body Play: The Book, Volume 1*, Menlo Park, CA, USA, 1995

Negri, Eve de, *Nigerian Body Adornment*, Lagos, 1976

Pasion, Dennie, *Making Faces*, London, 1999

Pepin Press, *Traditional Henna Designs*, Amsterdam, 2000

Perutz, Kathrin, *Beyond the Looking Glass: Life in the Beauty Culture*, Harmondsworth, UK, 1972 (2nd edn)

Peterkin, Allan, *One Thousand Beards: A Cultural History of Facial Hair*, Vancouver, 2001

Phaidon Press, *Fruits*, London, 2001

Polhemus, Ted, *Body Art: The Total Guide to Body Decoration*, Shaftesbury, UK, 1998

Polhemus, Ted, *Bodystyles*, Luton, UK, 1988

Polhemus, Ted (ed.), *Social Aspects of the Human Body*, Harmondsworth, UK, 1978

Polhemus, Ted, *Streetstyle: From Sidewalk to Catwalk*, London, 1997 (2nd edn)

Polhemus, Ted, *Style Surfing: What to Wear in the 3rd Millennium*, London, 1996

Polhemus, Ted and Lynn Procter, *Fashion & Anti-Fashion: An Anthropology of Clothing and Adornment*, London, 1978

Polhemus, Ted and Housk Randall, *The Customized Body*, London, 2000 (2nd edn)

Poppi, Cesare, 'The Other Within: Masks and Masquerades in Europe' in John Mack (ed.) *Masks and the Art of Expression*, London, 1994

Ragas, Meg Cohen and Karen Kozlowski, *Read My Lips: A Cultural History of Lipstick*, San Francisco, 1998

Randall, Housk, *Revelations*, London, 1993

RE/Search Publications, *Modern Primitives: An Investigation of Contemporary Adornment and Ritual*, Eugene, USA, 1989 (3rd edn)

Richie, Donald and Ian Buruma, *The Japanese Tattoo*, New York, 1982 (2nd edn)

Richter, Stefan, *Tattoo*, London, 1985

Riefenstahl, Leni, *The Last of the Nuba*, London, 1986 (4th edn)

Roberts, Allen F., 'Tabwa Tegumentary Inscription' in Arnold Rubin (ed.) *Marks of Civilization*, Los Angeles, 1988, pp. 41–56

Robinson, Julian, *Body Packaging: A Guide to Human Sexual Display*, Los Angeles, 1988

Robinson, Julian, *The Quest for Human Beauty*, New York, 1998

Robley H. G., *Moko: The Art and History of Maori Tattooing*, Twickenham, UK, 1998 (first published London, 1896)

Rubin, Arnold (ed.), *Marks of Civilization*, Los Angeles, 1988

Rudofsky, Bernard, *The Unfashionable Human Body*, London, 1972

Sagay, Esi, *African Hairstyles: Styles of Yesterday and Today*, Oxford, 1983

Saint-Laurent, Cecil, *The Great Book of Lingerie*, London, 1986

Schiffmacher, Henk, *1,000 Tattoos*, Cologne, 1996

Scutt, Ronald and Christopher Gotch, *Skin Deep: The Mystery of Tattooing*, London, 1974

Shelton, Anthony, 'Fictions and Parodies: Masquerade in Mexico and Highland South America' in John Mack (ed.) *Masks and the Art of Expression*, London, 1994

Spindler, Konrad, *The Man in the Ice*, London, 1995 (2nd edn)

Sinclair, N., *The Chameleon Body*, London, 1996

Steffen, Alfred, *Portrait of a Generation: The Love Parade Family Book*, Cologne, 1997

Stoddart, D. Michael, *The Scented Ape: The Biology and Culture of Human Odour*, Cambridge, 1990

Strathern, Andrew and Marilyn, *Self-Decoration in Mount Hagen*, London, 1971

Tanizaki, Junichirō, *In Praise of Shadows*, London, 2001

Tattersall, Ian, *The Monkey in the Mirror: Essays on the Science of What Makes Us Human*, New York, 2002

Thévoz, Michel, *The Painted Body*, Geneva, 1984

Thomas, Nicholas, *Oceanic Art*, London, 1995

Thomson, R. G., *Extraordinary Bodies: Figuring Physical Disability in American Culture and Literature*, New York, 1997

Thomson, R. G. (ed.), *Freakery: Cultural Spectacles of the Extraordinary Body*, New York, 1996

Trasko, Mary, *Daring Do's: A History of Extraordinary Hair*, Paris, 1994

Ucko, Peter J., 'Penis Sheaths: A Comparative Study' in *Proceedings of the Royal Anthropological Institute of Great Britain and Ireland for 1969*, London, 1970, pp. 27–68

Verswijver, Gustaaf, *Mekranoti: Living Among the Painted People of the Amazon*, Munich, 1996

Violette Editions, *Leigh Bowery*, London, 1998

Virel, André, *Decorated Man: The Human Body as Art*, New York, 1980 (2nd edn)

Vogel, Susan, 'Baule Scarification: The Mark of Civilization', in Arnold Rubin (ed.) *Marks of Civilization*, Los Angeles, 1988, pp. 97–106

Wakefield, Neville, *Postmodernism: The Twilight of the Real*, London, 1990

Walgrave, Jan, *The Ego Adorned: 20th-Century Artists' Jewellery*, Antwerp, 2000

Willem, G., *Irezumi: The Pattern of Dermatography in Japan*, Leiden, 1982

Willett, Frank, *African Art*, London, 1971

Wood, David T. G. (ed.), *Body Probe: Mutating Physical Boundaries*, London, 1999

Woodforde, John, *The Strange Story of False Hair*, London, 1971

Wroblewski, Chrisotpher, *Skin Show: The Art and Craft of Tattoo*, Leicester, 1981

FURTHER INFORMATION

WEBSITES & MAGAZINES

www.amnh.org/exhibitions/bodyart
[American Museum of Natural History, 'Body Art: Marks of Identity' > an anthropological overview]

www.amonline.net.au/bodyart
[Australian Museum> useful sections on face/body painting, piercing, scarification, tattooing, shaping the body, henna, etc.]

www.beautyworlds.com
[historical, anthropological and practical info. on hairstyling and cosmetics]

www.blackhairmedia.com
[practical advice and ideas for hairstyling and cosmetics]

www.bmezine.com
[comprehensive body modification ezine with subsections on piercing, scarification, tattooing, etc., some adult material]

www.bodyart.com
[links to hundreds of specialist sites on body decoration and modification, often with practical advice]

www.body-art.net
['No Body Is Perfect'; beautifully designed and photographed, with emphasis on highly adventurous new directions in body decoration/ modification, strong adult content]

www.bodyplay.com
[once a printed magazine, this is the site of seminal Modern Primitive Fakir Musafar; anthropological background and practical guide to what some will consider extreme body modifications and ritual practices, some adult material]

http://energytat2.com
[beautifully designed site featuring the distinctive tattoo art of Punko, Barcelona]

www.ethnicarts.org/body arts
[links site for piercing, tattoos, henna and masks]

www.galerie-ra.nl
[beautifully designed site which features work by many of today's most interesting contemporary jewelry designers]

www.hennapage.com
[history and practical advice on henna]

www.keibunsha.com
[Japan Tattoo Institute > info. and images of Japanese tattooing]

www.mehndiskinart.com
[henna designs, artists and products]

www.museum.upenn.edu/new/ exhibits/online_exhibits/body-modification
[Penn University Museum > anthropological perspective]

www.nailartgallery.com
[new designs in nail art]

www.newyorkadorned.com
[New York Adorned Studio > showcase of piercings, henna, jewelry and tattooing]

www.quinnster.co.uk
[everything you ever wanted to know about hair extensions]

www.safepiercing.org
[Association of Professional Piercers (US) > practical health advice on piercing]

www.schmucksymposium.de
[info. about the annual Zimmerhof jewelry design conference, which brings together many of the best in this field, in German, English version in preparation]

http//tattoo.about.com/cs/beginners/1/blsiteatoz.htm
[extensive practical guide to body piercing, scarification, henna and tattooing, and various tattoo styles]

www.tattooarchive.com
[a–z archive of tattoo history]

www.tattooheaven.com
[extraordinarily comprehensive studies of both ancient and contemporary tattooing. Also some material on henna, kohl, scarification and branding]

www.tattoos.com
[comprehensive review of tattoo world including style galleries and an a–z of studios]

www.tattoostudioguide.com
[tattoo studios and styles in the UK]

www.tattootraditions.alohaworld.com
[photos and text about tattooing in the Pacific]

www.tedpolhemus.com
[the author's site, which includes sections on body decoration, streetstyle and style as communication]

www.triangletattoo.com
['Art With A Pulse'; including info on Triangle Tattoo and Museum in Ft. Bragg, CA, USA]

www.tribalectic.com/EZine.asp
[piercing discussion, practical info and picture gallery]

www.vanishingtattoo.com
[fantastic virtual tour of tattooing in Borneo, Japan, Polynesia, China, Russia and elsewhere plus contemporary designs, practical advice, books, etc.]

Black Beauty and Hair
Hawker Consumer Publications Ltd, 2nd fl. Culvert House, Culvert Rd, Battersea, London SW11 5DH, UK, www.blackbeautyandhair.com

Black Hair
Freebournes House, Freebournes Rd, Witham, Essex CM8 3US, UK

Cutie
[Japanese streetstyle magazine]
Takarajima Corporation, Ichban-Chiyou -25, Chiyoda-Ku, Tokyo 102-8388, Japan

Estetica
[International hairstyling magazine]
1 Maple St, Unit 8A, East Rutherford, NJ 07073, USA]

Fruits
[Japanese streetstyle magazine]
Street Henshu Shitu Company, 1-16-8-5F, Ebisu Nishi, Shibya-Ku, Tokyo 150-0021 Japan

Hair Now
109/110 Bolsover St, London W1W 5NT, UK

Internationnal Tattoo Art
Butterfly Publications, 462 Broadway, 4th floor, New York, NY 10013, USA

In the Skin
Outlaw Biker Enterprises, 5 Marineview Plaza, no.207, Hoboken, NJ 07030, USA

Make-up Artist Magazine
P. O. Box 4316 Sunland, CA 91041-4316, USA, www.make-upmag.com

Passion
[International hairstyling magazine]
Dowa Planning Inc., Dairoku Seiko Bldg., 1-31 Akassaka, 5-chrome, Minato-ku, Tokyo 107, Japan

Skin and Ink
LFP Inc., 8484 Wilshire Blvd., Suite 900, Beverly Hills, CA 90211, USA

Skin Deep
P. O. Box 23619, London E7 9TY, UK, www.skindeep.co.uk

Skin Shots
P. O. Box 23619, London E7 9TY, UK, www.skinshots.co.uk

Skin Two
[Fetish style magazine]
Tim Woodward Publishing Ltd, 63 Abbey Business Centre, Ingate Pl., London SW8 3NS, UK

Tattoo
Paisano Publications, 28210 Dorothy Dr., Agoura Hills, CA 19301, USA

Tattoo Energy
Via De Amicis 35, 20123 Milan, Italy www.tattoolife.com

Tattoo Flash
Paisano Publications, 28210 Dorothy Dr., Agoura Hills, CA 19301, USA

Tattoo Life
Via De Amicis 35, 20123 Milan, Italy, www.tattoolife.com

Tattoo Savage
Paisano Publications, 28210 Dorothy Dr., Agoura Hills, CA 19301, USA

ACKNOWLEDGMENTS

Every effort has been made to trace the copyright holders of the images and designs contained in this book, and we apologize in advance for any unintentional omissions. We would be pleased to insert the appropriate acknowledgment in any subsequent edition of this publication.

cover & p. 6 Maud
styling: Stainless Sharon at Dare 2 Wear

pp. 8–9 & back cover Grace & Tory, p. 19 Elisa & Elisa, p. 98 Kirsten, Marina
from the series '7–11' for
Pulp Magazine, Belgium
model: Marina at Touché
styling: Berber de Jong
make-up: Stainless Sharon at Dare2Wear
hair: Taco at House of Orange
extensions: Purple Circle

p. 20 Barbara
make-up: Claudette

pp. 24–25 Valesca, Isabella
make-up: Nise

pp. 26, 128–129 & 131 Martin
thanks to Max Models
hair & make-up: Dino

pp. 35 & 37 Etsuko, p. 36 Joyce & Priscilla
thanks to Kitseroo
styling: Kik at Poe
make-up: Dino

pp. 45 & 115 Marc
tattoos by: Damon from Perth, WA;
Locky Lawrence at W. A. Ink, Fremantle, Perth, W.A.; Ernesto at Borneo Headhunters, Borneo; Jeroen Franken formerly at Hanky Panky, Amsterdam; Eddie and Simon Umpie at Borneo Ink, Kuala Lumpur; Steve Cross at Tattoo Connection, Melbourne, Australia; Ibans of Lalang, Skrang River, Sarawak, Borneo

pp. 84–85 Nadia, p. 137 Iris
from the series 'Abduction'
model: Iris at de Boekers
make-up: Mascha at House of Orange

p. 86 Marie-Louise
from the series 'Body Snatchers'
for *Basic Groove Magazine*, Netherlands
styling: Lee
make-up: Dino
hair: Arjan

p. 92 Sonny, Jenny-Li
thanks to anti-models.nl

p. 97 Vianney
from the series 'Profile' for
Stick Magazine, Sweden
model: Vianney at de Boekers
make-up: Benjamin Puckey at House of Orange
hair: Rutger at House of Orange

p. 97 Giovanca
from the series 'Colorifique'
model: Giovanca at AFT
hair & make-up: Taco at House of Orange

p. 98 Anja
make-up: Stainless Sharon at Dare2Wear

pp. 134–135 & 137 D-Monica & Chico
hair & make-up: Stainless Sharon at Dare2Wear

Thanks to the following studios:

PIERCING & TATTOOS
Admiraal Tattoo
Marnixstraat 151, 1015 VM Amsterdam, the Netherlands
t +31 (0) 20 6223218
e info@admiraaltattoo.com
www.admiraaltattoo.com

Anjelique Houtkamp Tattooing
Amsterdam, the Netherlands
www.salonserpent.com

Dare2Wear Body Piercing
Buiten Oranjestraat 15, 1013 HX, Amsterdam, the Netherlands
t +31 (0) 20 686 8679
www.dare2wear.info

Eyegasm Tattoo
Kerkstraat 113, Amsterdam, the Netherlands
t +31 (0) 20 330 3767
www.eyegasm.org

Fox Tattoo
Paardensteeg 6, 3441 TN Woerden, the Netherlands
t +31 (0) 34 868 9066
e info@foxtattoo.nl
www.foxtattoo.nl

Henna Tattoo by Danny
Amsterdam, the Netherlands
t +31 (0) 6 25124889

The Inkstitution
Schiewg 141a, 3038 AN Rotterdam, the Netherlands
t +31 (0) 10 4666747
e inkstitution@yahoo.com,
www.inkstitution.com

ORNAMENTS & JEWELRY
Allycat Jewellery at Cyberdog
The Stables Market, Chalk Farm Rd, London NW1, UK
e allycatfetishwear@blueyonder.co.uk

Cyberdog
The Stables Market, Chalk Farm Rd, London NW1, UK
t +44 (0) 20 7482 2842
e info@cyberdog.net
www.cyberdog.net

Galerie Ra
Vijzel Straat 80,
1017 HL Amsterdam, the Netherlands
t +31 (0) 20 626 5100
e mail@galerie-ra.nl
www.galerie-ra.nl

Medusa Gothic Party Amsterdam
www.medusa-amsterdam.nl

Pet Salon Millinery
Amsterdam, the Netherlands

SPECIALIST HAIRDRESSING
Pepi's Hairspace
Unit 33, The Stables Market, Chalk Farm Rd,
London NW1 8AH, UK
t +44 (0) 20 7485 5266
e londonpepis@hotmail.com
www.head-space.org/Pepis

Emm & Bees Hair2Do
Tube 2, The Stables Market, Chalk Farm Rd,
London NW1 9LQ, UK
t +44 (0) 20 7485 5318
e EmmandBees@aol.com

UZi PART B would like to dedicate this book to all those who freely and generously gave their time to pose for us, and to Stainless Sharon at Dare2Wear Piercing, Amsterdam, without whom there would be no Hot Bodies, Cool Styles.

Special thanks to Nick Strong
at Cheap 'n' Nasty Image Manipulation, Amsterdam
Thanks to Anja and everyone
at Cyberdog

Ted Polhemus would like to thank...

...for advice, information and encouragement:

Jewelry designers Florian Ladstätter [contact@ladstaetter.de], Naomi Filmer [naomi_filmer@mac.com], Masako Hamaguchi [masako@hamaguchi.demon.co.uk] and Paul Derrez at Galerie Ra, Amsterdam [www.galerie-ra.nl]

Singer, writer and arts/style consultant Carol Leeming of Nia & Dare To Diva Productions [iriediva@hotmail.com]

Anthropologist Ellisiv Flatval [flatval@stud.ntnu.no]

Clothing designer and fashion illustrator Carol Ryder of Carol Ryder Clothing Design and Illustration [carol@carolryder.co.uk, www.carolryder.co.uk]

Photographer and dancer Mrs Love at (together with Betti Marenko) in.sect.corp [mrslove@quattro.co.za, www.mrslove.org, www.insectcorp.com]

Body modifier and tattooist Dave Tusk of Tusk Tatoo [info@tusktattoo.com, www.tusktattoo.com]

Publisher Miki Vialetto at *Tattoo Life Magazine* [mikivialetto@planet.it, www.tattoolife.com]

Tattooists Bugs at Evil from the Needle, London [info@bugsart.co.uk, www.bugsart.co.uk] and Alex Binnie at Into You, London [a.binnie@virgin.net, www.into-you.co.uk]

...the tattoo artists who provided samples of their artwork for reproduction in this book, and their studios:

Andi Bone
Tribalize
30 Lower Marsh,
London SE1 7RG, UK
t +44 (0) 20 7928 1231

Alex Binnie, Jason Saga
and Xed le Head
Into You
144 St John's St,
London EC1, UK
t +44 (0) 20 7253 5085
www.into-you.co.uk

Bugs
Evil from the Needle
232 Camden High Street,
London NW1 8QS, UK
t +44 (0) 20 7482 2414
info@bugsart.co.uk
www.bugsart.co.uk

Matt Differ
Tusk Tattoo & Body Piercing
1 Stukeley St,
London WC2B 5LB, UK
t +44 (0) 20 7404 5999
info@tusktattoo.com
www.tusktattoo.com

Michelle Myles
Dare Devil Tattoo
174 Ludlow St, NYC,
NY 10002, USA
t +1 212 533 8303
Daredevil1nyc@aol.com
www.daredeviltattooing.com

Yorg (George Powell)
Medusa Tattoo
85 Kallidromiou/Exarcheia,
10683 Athens, Greece
t +30 210 8254 593
yorgtat@hotmail.com
www.medusatattoo.com

Amanda Toy and Rudy Fritsch
Original Classic Tattoo
Via Diaz 221E, 34100 Trieste, Italy
t +39 040 313130
amanda.toy@originalclassictattoo.com
rudy.fritsch@originalclassictattoo.com
www.originalclassictattoo.com